Wolfberry

Nature's Bounty of Nutrition & Health

To Dr. Joe Bissett
Best Wishes & Warmest Regards

Frank Tompkin
4-2-2010

Paul M. Gross, PhD,
Xiaoping Zhang, MD,
Richard Zhang

WOLFBERRY
Nature's Bounty of Nutrition & Health

2006

Wolfberry

Nature's Bounty of Nutrition & Health

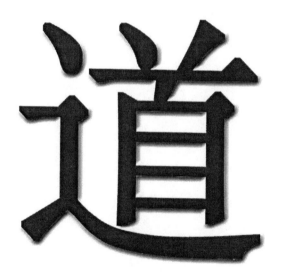

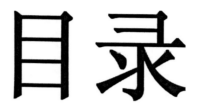

Wolfberry

Nature's Bounty of Nutrition & Health

TABLE OF CONTENTS

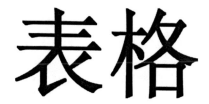

INDEX OF TABLES

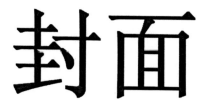

FRONT COVER

The brilliance of Ningxia wolfberries is contrasted against the barren Loess Plateau and Huang He (Yellow River, lower) in the background. Photo from Jingtai, Gansu; credit, Prof. George Leung, University of Massachusetts, Dartmouth.

Mineral-rich dust formed by glaciation 2 million years ago—the loess of Ningxia's western neighbor, Gansu Province—is wind-eroded into the river basin where the Huang He, named for its yellow loessal color, carries sediment downstream into Ningxia.

The most silt-laden river in the world, Huang He has flooded annually over centuries, depositing silt onto Ningxia's riverside plains. The flood sediments create ideal soil fertility for Ningxia's famous premium wolfberries to absorb loessal nutrients, no doubt a significant factor in wolfberry's nutritional content.

致献

Dedication

Our book is dedicated to the memory and work of Cui Yueli, MD (1920-1998), Chinese Minister of Health from 1978 to 1987. Dr. Cui dedicated his life to the heritage and development of traditional Chinese medicine (TCM) in China.

TCM was the mainstream healthcare system in China before the 1930s but became ignored or actively banned for decades thereafter. When the communist party gained power in 1949, China adopted the western and Soviet medical care systems that spread across the country over the next 40 years. TCM practice was still neglected until the middle 1980s when Dr. Cui realized he needed to actively promote TCM to preserve this 5,000 year old treasure.

After medical training in the Chinese military, Dr. Cui Yueli developed a great passion toward TCM. During two terms of service in the Chinese Ministry of Health, Dr. Cui convinced the government to invest hundreds of millions of Chinese yuan to preserve TCM, support its clinics, and form a State Bureau for TCM.

As Health Minister, Dr. Cui engineered expansion of TCM clinics from 100 to several thousand countrywide in 1990. He urged hospitals to provide space for TCM doctors and support scientific research on Chinese herbs as medicines, giving new life to the ancient traditions. Dr. Cui met personally with countless young physicians, encouraging them to study from traditional TCM masters and incorporate TCM knowledge into their conventional medical practices. This helped to establish the new field of integrative medicine blending TCM with modern western medical knowledge. Over the 1980s and 90s, Dr. Cui Yueli became the most respected medical officer in China and was truly loved by TCM industry leaders and practitioners throughout the world, as his memory remains today.

To sustain respect for TCM and encourage introduction of China's herbal treasures to the United States, Dr. Cui asked his daughter, Dr. Xiaoping Zhang, and Richard Zhang—coauthors of this book—to form a company facilitating access to Chinese herbal products with TCM applications. The wolfberry is renowned to have this use as an herbal medicine over the course of Chinese recorded history.

In 1998, Rich Nature Nutraceutical Laboratories, Inc. was established in Seattle.

When Dr. Cui passed away in 1998, the China Bureau of TCM supported formation of the Cui Yueli TCM Research Center in Beijing where the science of herbal medicines is being studied today in a variety of basic and clinical research programs.

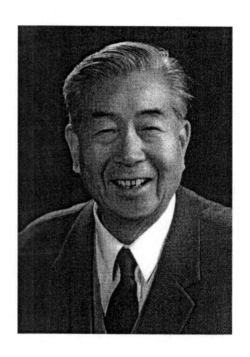

Dr. Cui Yueli (1920-1998)

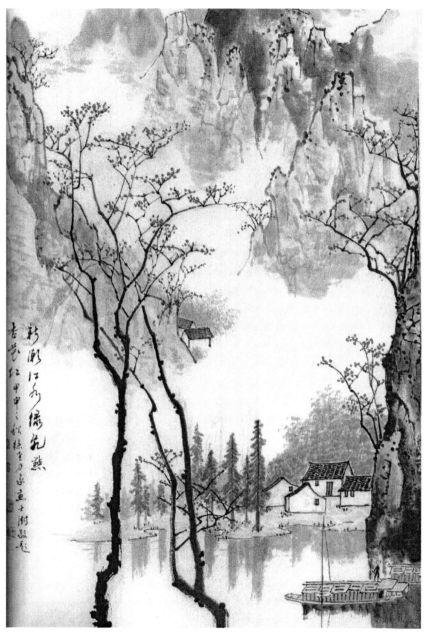

"Village River", ink on xuan paper (1998) by Ms. Xu Shulin, wife of
Dr. Cui Yueli, mother of Dr. Xiaoping Zhang (co-author of this book),
former Director of the Beijing Opera, now living in Beijing.

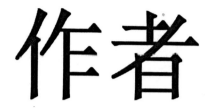

AUTHOR BIOGRAPHIES

Dr. Paul M. Gross received his PhD degree in Physiology from the University of Glasgow, Scotland and was trained in neuroscience at the National Institutes of Health, Bethesda, Maryland. A Canadian, he was a Research Scholar of the Heart and Stroke Foundation of Ontario and recipient of the Heinz Karger Memorial Award, Switzerland, for publications on brain capillaries. Dr. Gross is a freelance science writer living on Vancouver Island, British Columbia.

Dr. Xiaoping Zhang received her MD degree from Beijing Medical University, trained as a resident in family medicine and was a general practice physician in China before moving to the United States. For 4 years in China, she received special training in traditional Chinese medicine. Dr. Zhang has a Master's degree in Public Health from the University of Hawaii and is co-founder of Rich Nature Nutraceutical Labs in Seattle where she now lives.

Richard Zhang was a medical information specialist at Hunan Medical University in China before attending the University of Hawaii where he received his Master's degree in Information Science. Mr. Zhang lives in Seattle and has promoted information about wolfberries in the United States since 1999. He owns a wolfberry farm in Zhongning County, Ningxia, China and is co-founder of Rich Nature Nutraceutical Labs.

感谢

ACKNOWLEDGEMENTS

We are grateful for friends who offered comments on the manuscript—Ted Fogg particularly, not only for editorial suggestions but for lessons on wolfberry farming and facilitating Amy Qi Lu to translate the Chinese horticultural sections in Chapter 9.

Dr. Dietmar Breithaupt, Stuttgart, Germany, Dr. Ron Wrolstad, Corvallis, Oregon, and Dr. Rong Cao, Guelph, Ontario each provided valuable critiques of scientific sections. Dr. Tom Gordon and Tina Harrower made helpful suggestions on organization. We thank Janie Hibler, author of *The Berry Bible,* for inspiration and sharing insights on her writing and publishing experiences.

We especially thank Dr. G. (Joe) Mazza, Summerland, British Columbia, for generous discussions about berry nutrients and functional foods.

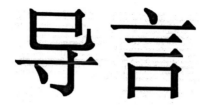

CHAPTER 1
Introduction

Is Wolfberry Nature's Most Nutritious Food?

What is it about the highest order of a species or landmark—the largest mammal (blue whale), highest mountain (Everest), or greatest golfer (Tiger Woods)—that seizes our attention and stirs our wonder?

We begin to think about qualities that set it apart from its competitors and so begin to define the origin, nature, values and potential of the greatest.

So it is with wolfberries, a fruit largely unknown in many first-world countries, but whose history in its native land of China is so profound that it is revered as a national treasure and perhaps the most nutritious food on Earth.

Presently in the United States and other prosperous western countries, a growing crisis of obesity and related diseases (diabetes, heart disease, hypertension, chronic inflammation) is looming. Inactive lifestyles combined with diets high in portions and low in nutrients cross age groups and social status.

Recognizing this trend, expert nutritionists are focusing the public's attention more on whole foods as solutions for comprehensive nutrient intake—that is, foods with multiple nutrients in a convenient single serving.

Having one food source provide many of the day's essential nutrients and calories would be an obvious advantage for simplifying good dietary practices—as long as it was combined with other selections from the Food Pyramid.

So we might naturally ask: what is Nature's most nutrient-dense food that can offer this advantage?

We can define high nutrient density as nutrient richness, or to say simply, the most nutrients in one serving. By then identifying individual nutrients, we gain insights to a food's overall nutritive benefits and the potential synergy nutrients have together.

Accordingly, this book was written to give nutritional background on wolfberry and present an objective view on the question introducing this chapter—is it the World's most nutrient-packed food?

Wolfberries might have one of the longest recorded traditions as a health food. They have been eaten as a favored snack and ingredient in various recipes with health benefits over 5,000 years of recorded Chinese history.

It is said the name wolfberry comes from ancient Chinese legends of the animal on top of the wild food chain across the plains and forests of old China—the omnivorous wolf—often seen engorging on ripe berries and leaves among the dense vines.

In more modern times, wolfberry fit as a name when it became known in China as the "alpha" food of nutritional herbs, i.e., like the alpha leader of the wolf pack, a higher nutrient density may not exist among plants.

The book was written to bring together available scientific evidence for wolfberry as a nutrient-dense food, as best as current information allows for a plant mostly unknown outside China where 99% of the world's commercial supply grows.

If eventually confirmed this way, wolfberry may gain acceptance as a healthy addition to diets in western countries now opening their markets to Chinese exports. Or it may eventually become a cultivated crop in amounts sufficient to supply one country's own demands for a nutrient-rich, delicious fruit that can contribute to healthier nutrition and lifestyles.

To help establish background, we present in the book a total of 81 research publications specifically pertaining to the wolfberry or its nutrients. We discuss nutritional classes to which wolfberry's special nutrients belong, how they compare with other nutrient-rich foods, and what diseases wolfberry nutrients may actually benefit.

Another goal is to provide varied background about the wolfberry plant. We give accounts of the legendary history, traditional Chinese medicine, botanical taxonomy, cultivation, harvesting and growing regions, soil factors and environmental conditions, effects of processing the fruit, and medical abstracts proposing wolfberry with a broad assortment of health benefits.

Our goal is to make wolfberry better understood outside SE Asia where it has lived in legend for thousands of years, revered as a king of medicinal plants rich in healthful nutrients.

***

At the time of proofreading the final manuscript in March 2006, we discovered publication of a new book on wolfberries by Gary Young, Ronald Lawrence and Marc Schreuder, entitled *Discovery of the Ultimate Superfood*, 2005, Essential Science Publishing, Orem, UT, ISBN 0-943685-44-3

植化

CHAPTER 2
Wolfberry Phytochemicals
What are Wolfberries?

Before we begin our examination of wolfberry nutrients, we want to fix a mental picture of this unique berry. On the front and back covers are pictures of wolfberries that we use as reminders of its characteristics while we move through the book. Sections later (Chapters 8,9) give more details about factors affecting wolfberry nutrients, such as its botanical family, soil and climate conditions, geographical harvesting regions, cultivation methods and other horticultural features.

Botanically, wolfberry belongs to the Solanaceae ("sole-an-eh-see-eye") family, also referred to as nightshades or boxthorns. By scientific or Latin designation, it is called *Lycium barbarum L.* "Lycium", the genus name, is thought to be from the ancient Mid-Asian geographic region of Lydia; barbarum, the species name, says its origin was "foreign" (perhaps external to China), and "L." indicates the name derived from the Linnaeus taxonomy format.

The name for wolfberry in Mandarin Chinese is gou qi zi where "zi" means berry. By colloquial practice, the name has sometimes become abbreviated further to "goji" berry.

There are hundreds of nightshade plants in the large Solanaceae family, such as the tomato, potato, tobacco and petunia, so one can see that wolfberry fits into a plant group providing edible fruit from colorful leafy blossoms. In the genus of this species, Lycium, are dozens of plants (see Chapter 8) yielding berries on boxthorn or matrimony vines, some of them poisonous.

Wolfberry fruit, growing along branches of these 3-15 ft vines, is a berry oblong in shape, bright red at full maturity and very juicy (front cover). Along the banks of China's Yellow River thousands of years ago when it was first documented as a favored food, wolfberries must have been a very tempting and easy to pick prize for travelers and early farmers.

Phytochemicals as Nutrients

Several factors must come together to endow an edible plant with high nutrition as wolfberry is reputed to have. These would include its phylogeny (or plant "family tree") determining its genetic endowment, environmental conditions of soil, weather, growing season, exposure to pests, cultivation methods and so on.

All these factors merge in wolfberry to establish a unique nutrient profile. A plant such as wolfberry may contain a variety of nutrients including those chemicals unique to its own makeup, giving it nutrient "signatures" that stand out among other berries or any edible plant. As we discuss later, wolfberry's signature nutrients are two classes of interesting and health-promoting phytochemicals—polysaccharide sugars (Chapter 4) and carotenoid pigments (Chapter 5).

A relatively new term in nutrition research is called "phytochemical" which means "plant-derived" chemical. Wolfberry is a fruit packed with phytochemicals, likely dozens of them in every berry. When nutritional properties are eventually known, phytochemicals will be referred to as phytonutrients.

And that is the primary goal of this book—to identify, organize and substantiate the scientific basis for wolfberry's great variety of phytochemicals that serve as nutrients.

Not only in plants are there large or "macro" nutrient classes in gram quantities like carbohydrates, proteins, fiber and fat but also smaller amounts of "micro" nutrients in milligram or microgram quantities. These include vitamins, minerals, amino acids and interesting groups of other promising chemicals such as carotenoids, phenolics, phytoestrogens, fatty acids and sterols.

Let's gain some perspective on phytochemicals from the Position

Statement of the American Dietetic Association, 1995, entitled *Phytochemicals and Functional Foods*

> *In addition to the nutrients that are involved in normal metabolic activity, foods contain components that may provide additional health benefits. These food components (generally referred to as phytochemicals) are derived from naturally occurring ingredients and are actively being investigated for their health-promoting potential. Health benefits of these foods are best obtained through the consumption of a varied diet using our normal food supply.*
>
> *These phytochemicals and/or health-preserving elements are present in a number of frequently consumed foods, especially fruits, vegetables, grains, legumes, and seeds, and in a number of less frequently consumed foods such as licorice, soy, and green tea. In addition, functional foods, which are defined as any modified food or food ingredient that may provide a health benefit beyond the traditional nutrients it contains, are being developed and subjected to scientific evaluation. In recent years, the number of functional foods that have potential benefits for health has grown tremendously. Scientific evidence is accumulating to support the role of phytochemicals and functional foods in the prevention and treatment of disease.*

The benefits of phytochemicals and functional foods have been extensively publicized in the popular press, resulting in increased public awareness and interest in consumption of phytochemical-rich foods and functional foods as a method of enhancing health and well-being. Although scientific evidence of clinical benefits is limited, evidence is mounting to support the incorporation of foods rich in phytochemicals into the diets of most Americans.

Although other accounts of phytochemical values to health have been published since 1995, this ADA advisory gives us good background for understanding the place in our diets for natural products like wolfberries.

It's valuable, therefore, to consider nutrients and phytochemicals of wolfberries as available science allows. That is the goal of this and following chapters as we begin to unravel wolfberry's nutrient profile.

Science-based guidelines for all phytochemical intake levels are not yet fully established although there are now government and expert panel advisories on intakes for vitamins, minerals and fiber. Watchdogs for public consumption of foods and specific nutrients, e.g., the US Department of Agriculture, US Food and Drug Administration, or Health Canada as western examples, have not yet published intake guidelines for all phytochemicals, saying there is insufficient research upon which to make recommendations.

This means science and clinical research have not yet laid sufficient foundation for the long-term benefits of phytochemicals, even if we do have growing evidence for the values of including more phytochemicals in our diets. As a result, their intake has not yet been defined as "essential" in the diet.

Excellent guidelines in popular media are emerging, however. One with relevance and background for this discussion of wolfberries is the 2004 book by Steven Pratt, MD and Kathy Matthews, *SuperFoods Rx*, describing 14 superfoods easily found in grocery store produce sections. As we'll see later in our discussion, the Pratt and Matthews information on blueberries, spinach and flax seeds as common superfoods gives great background for better understanding wolfberries or any nutrient-rich food.

There may be as many as 8,000 individual phytochemicals among natural foods, with dozens occurring in a single nutrient-dense plant like the flax seed or wolfberry. These chemicals are more than just calories, vitamins, minerals or fatty acids—some are simple pigments that may offer broad health benefits preventing or delaying onset of diseases and effects of aging.

Simply with that message is a glimpse of why wolfberries have been popular in China for dozens of centuries and why we are motivated to write this book.

One fact from nutrition research on phytochemicals is clear, however. Consumption of the *whole* food (or perhaps a comprehensive nutritional supplement) guarantees intake of as many of the intact phytonutrients as possible. Once inside our bodies, the macro- and micronutrients can act in concert and so complement one another, a process some nutritionists refer to as *nutritional synergy*.

Such synergy may in fact explain wolfberry's numerous potential health benefits. For example, wolfberry's famous polysaccharide sugars are not only immunologically active (Chapter 4). They are also a major source of dietary soluble fiber that may

1)   enhance calcium, magnesium and iron absorption,

2)   help stabilize blood glucose (sugar) levels after a meal,

3)   contribute to lowering blood cholesterol,

4)   promote colon health by increasing production of fatty acids and raising acidity levels, thereby reducing colon cancer risk and

5)   afford immune protection through a comprehensive array of intermediate effects within the intestinal system.

We'll devote more attention to synergy later in this chapter.

Until we have the full story about such minute interactions between numerous phytonutrients in a single food like wolfberry, one conclusion seems clear—the safest and most effective way to benefit from wolfberry's bounty of nutrients is to eat the whole fruit, including its skin and seeds. We will need to consider, therefore, that the wolfberry juice products popularized on the internet and through multi-level marketing companies may omit beneficial phytonutrients left behind in the pomace from the juicing process (Chapter 10).

Another factor we'll consider in Chapter 10 is the processing of a multinutrient source like wolfberry for its individual extracts. Treatment of fruit pulp with solvents like alcohol, acetone, mild acids, heat and even simple mechanical methods can de-nature and/or diminish amounts of phytochemicals.

Simply, processing of a fruit to powder or juice may reduce its overall phytochemical value by minimizing the nutritional importance of skin and seeds. Eating the whole fresh or dried fruit likely provides optimal benefits.

Phytochemicals for Health

Medical studies to date have demonstrated that phytochemicals in common fruits and vegetables can have overlapping mechanisms of action, including such beneficial effects as

•   antioxidant activity and scavenging free radicals

•   regulation of gene expression in cell reproduction and repair, cell differentiation, and stimulation of cancer and tumor-suppressor genes

- induction of normal and abnormal cell death mechanisms (apoptosis, pronounced "eh-poe-toe-sis")
- modulation of enzyme activities
- stimulation of immune system responses
- regulation of hormone metabolism
- antibacterial or antiviral mechanisms

As evident from this incomplete list, dietary phytochemicals enter into countless cell activities involved in moment-to-moment life and long-term health. To put it another way, ingestion of mixed phytochemicals through a diet of whole foods may be important to prevention of as many as 60 diseases related to the list above.

Why minimize such a valuable set of nutritional benefits by focusing on just one or a few extracts from a food source, as so many supplement products propose to do?

"Superfoods" as discussed by Pratt and Mathews have been given credit for providing all these health benefits in a convenient package *as the whole food*.

As we move through the book, we'll examine pertinent research publications and offer interpretations where science is adequate to support claims of whole food nutrient synergy and how wolfberries may supply this benefit.

Phytochemicals, Antioxidants and Cancer

Cells in humans and other organisms are constantly exposed to a variety of oxidizing agents, some of which are necessary for life. These agents may be present in air, food, and water, or they may be produced even by normal metabolic activity within our cells.

Some are called "free radicals" or specifically "radical oxygen species" (ROS), meaning a reactive chemical such as singlet oxygen (O_2) formed when one atom of oxygen leaves the stable gas, O_2. A key health factor is to maintain a delicate balance between oxidizing agents and food-derived antioxidants to sustain optimal physiological conditions in health.

Overproduction of oxidizing chemicals or leaving them unchecked due to poor nutrition can cause an imbalance, leading to a condition called *oxidative stress*, especially in chronic diseases. Oxidative stress can cause damage to cell components like lipids important in cell membranes, proteins, and cell DNA affecting our genes, resulting in an increased risk for cancer cell development and potential onset of other diseases.

To prevent or slow oxidative stress induced by free radicals, sufficient amounts of dietary antioxidants need to be consumed. Fruits, vegetables, whole grains, seeds and nuts contain a wide variety of antioxidant compounds, such as phenolic acids and carotenoid pigments (Chapter 5), that may help protect cellular systems from ROS and so lower risk of chronic diseases.

Medical research and nutritional studies have shown that regular consumption of fruits and vegetables can reduce cancer risk via these antioxidant mechanisms.

One analysis of some 200 epidemiological studies examined the relationship between intake of fruits and vegetables and cancer of the lung, colon, breast, cervix, esophagus, mouth and throat, stomach, bladder, pancreas, and ovary. The consumption of fruits and vegetables was found to have a significant protective effect on cancer development in these body organs.

Risk of cancer was higher in persons with a low intake of fruits and vegetables than in those with a high intake. Fruits were significantly protective in cancer of the esophagus, mouth, and larynx (throat). Combined fruit and vegetable intake was protective for cancer of the pancreas, stomach, colon and bladder.

The initiation of cancer is a multistep process and oxidative damage is linked to the formation of tumors through various mechanisms. Oxidative stress causes cell DNA damage, which if unrepaired, can lead to genetic mutations and cell structure breakdown or rearrangement of cell components. This potentially cancer-inducing oxidative damage might be prevented or limited by dietary antioxidants found in fruits and vegetables.

As we shall see in Chapters 4-6, wolfberries have been studied by Chinese scientists over the past 30 years as a possible preventative for these effects.

Antioxidants

We have mentioned the word "antioxidant", to be given more in depth coverage in Chapter 5, as this is an important phytochemical category thought to be a major characteristic of wolfberries.

What are antioxidants and their potential health benefits?

Antioxidants are substances synthesized in the body or obtained via food nutrients that can prevent or slow oxidative damage to our body's cells.

Scientists believe that plants make antioxidants especially as pigments in their fruit skin, rind and seeds to protect the plant's regenerative capacity from the damaging effects of constant exposure to sunlight, ultraviolet radiation, pests and oxygen.

Antioxidant phytochemicals such as blueberry anthocyanins contribute blue-purple pigment to the berry skin, and so play a useful role in attracting insect pollinators and birds that eat the fruit then disperse seeds in their droppings. Plants also would benefit from antioxidant protection in the skin against photo-oxidative processes, viral or bacterial pathogens, benefits that can be passed on to animals consuming the berry.

Without protective antioxidants from pigments like carotenoids and anthocyanins in plant skin, reactive oxygen species could be created during normal photosynthesis leading to oxidative injury to proteins, lipids and nucleic acids, alteration in gene transcription, and even programmed cell death ("apoptosis") in the fruit or its seeds. Some botanists and food chemists refer to this protective benefit as *"pigment power"* desirable to obtain through the diet. For humans, this occurs by eating colorful fruits, vegetables and animal sources and so gaining the benefits of pigment power.

When human cells use oxygen, they naturally produce free radicals as by-products of normal metabolism that can lead to cell damage if normal counter-balances are not present in the environment inside and around our cells.

Antioxidants synthesized internally or those we obtain from our diets act as neutralizing sponges or "free radical scavengers". They counterbalance, absorb, quench, prevent or repair damage done by free radicals. Health problems such as heart disease, hypertension, macular degeneration of the eyes, diabetes, cancer, and inflammation are influenced to some degree by oxidative damage and, apparently, by insufficient amounts of internal and dietary antioxidants.

As we study wolfberries and other fruit, vegetables and herbs with antioxidant properties, we shall see the enormous variety of antioxidant phytochemicals thought to number many thousands across the plant world.

Two classes that characterize darkly-colored berries, however, are the primary antioxidant class of phenolic acids or polyphenols, i.e., the numerous phenolic species common in blueberries, black raspberries, pomegranate and acai. Later in the book to provide simple terminology, we refer generally to all polyphenolic compounds as "phenolics".

Carotenoids, a separate phytochemical class providing intense antioxidant activity, are abundant in wolfberries, discussed in Chapter 5.

An example of the nutritional and anti-cancer values of antioxidants from the scientific literature:

Publication. J Nutr. 2004 Dec;134(12 Suppl):3479S-3485S. **Potential synergy of phytochemicals in cancer prevention: mechanism of action.** Liu RH.Department of Food Science, Cornell University, Ithaca, NY, USA.

Abstract. Epidemiological studies have consistently shown that regular consumption of fruits and vegetables is strongly associated with reduced risk of developing chronic diseases, such as cancer and cardiovascular disease. It is now widely believed that the actions of the antioxidant nutrients alone do not explain the observed health benefits of diets rich in fruits and vegetables, because taken alone, the individual antioxidants studied in clinical trials do not appear to have consistent preventive effects. Work performed by our group and others has shown that fruits and vegetable phytochemical extracts exhibit strong antioxidant and antiproliferative activities and that the major part of total antioxidant activity is from the combination of phytochemicals.

We proposed that *the additive and synergistic effects of phytochemicals in fruits and vegetables are responsible for these potent antioxidant and anticancer activities and that the benefit of a diet rich in fruits and vegetables is attributed to the complex mixture of phytochemicals present in whole foods.* This explains why no single antioxidant can replace the combination of natural phytochemicals in fruits and vegetables to achieve the health benefits. The evidence suggests that antioxidants or bioactive compounds are best acquired through whole food consumption.

Synopsis. Systematic studies of large groups of people allow inferences about population masses ("epidemiological studies" or "clinical trials"). These studies show that eating whole foods rich in antioxidant nutrients provides a "synergy" of benefits for reducing cancer risk.

Such information is supported by other authors with two points we emphasize in this book: 1) consumption of a whole fruit (or other food source rich in nutrients) is likely to confer the greatest nutritional benefit and 2) choice of high-nutrient, high-antioxidant foods can help establish a base for good lifelong nutrition and health (also see Pratt and Matthews, 2004).

As we hope to provide the reader with as much information about wolfberries as available in present literature, one goal is to methodically identify nutrients conferring potential health value (Chapters 3 and 6). We also wish to compare wolfberry's nutritional profile to those of other well known, nutrient-dense foods. Accordingly, the next chapter will be used to detail these nutrients and comparisons.

Wolfberry Nutrients and Possible Health Benefits

Wolfberry is a native Chinese plant used in traditional Chinese medicine for 5,000 years but with little international export until recently. As a result of this limited economy and lack of western science applied to wolfberry research, the plant is hardly known outside Asia. Exotic natural products from around the world are increasingly entering the mainstream of health foods in first-world countries so it is timely to consider nutritional benefits wolfberry may eventually offer to western diets.

Wolfberry fruit, seeds, leaves, roots and bark have been used by the Chinese for centuries in many herbal formulas to maintain overall health against fatigue, visual degeneration in aging, headaches, insomnia, inflammation, chronic liver diseases, diabetes, tuberculosis, hypertension and a host of other ailments outlined further in Chapters 6 and 7. For centuries, Chinese shamans and herbalists have advised use of wolfberry to make tea, soup, stew and wine or suggest chewing dried berries as snacks like raisins for daily maintenance of general health.

Legendary stories of its health benefits have established wolfberry as a Chinese national treasure revered over centuries as a fountain of youth.

What is known about wolfberry in the western world today, however, is mainly from unscientific misinformation published on the internet to promote juice products—Goji Juice and NingXia Red Juice (a product new in 2005 previously called Berry Young Juice).

Summarized from web publications by the two manufacturers are potential health benefits of wolfberry juice

1. Extends life, protects against premature aging, has powerful antioxidant actions
2. Increases energy and strength
3. Stimulates secretion of human growth hormone and promotes youthful appearance
4. Maintains healthy blood pressure
5. Reduces blood cholesterol levels
6. Promotes normal blood sugar levels in diabetes mellitus
7. Enhances sexual functions and improves fertility
8. Helps lose weight
9. Relieves headaches and dizziness
10. Relieves insomnia
11. Supports eye health
12. Strengthens the heart and cardiovascular system
13. Improves disease resistance, strengthens immune responses, protects cellular DNA
14. Builds strong blood
15. Supports a healthy liver and pancreas
16. Treats menopausal symptoms
17. Prevents morning sickness during the early phase of pregnancy
18. Strengthens muscles and bones
19. Improves memory
20. Supports normal kidney function
21. Relieves chronic cough
22. Alleviates anxiety and stress
23. Promotes cheerfulness

What a list of possible benefits from the juice of just one fruit! It is likely, however, that these anticipated health benefits were extrapolated from findings of preliminary Chinese research or traditional Chinese practices where the whole fruit was used in diets and remedies. Observations on just a few people may have been magnified to infer large-scale comprehensive benefits. Consequently, we need to inspect that background carefully and objectively, a goal of this book.

Let's note that NingXia Red Juice (a wolfberry puree of berry pulp, skin, seeds and stem) is made to include juices of other nutritional berry fruits, such as the popular and scientifically validated blueberry and pomegranate. NingXia Red also contains orange and lemon essential oils, both of which contribute potent antioxidant qualities. A 2005 booklet by H. Rodier, MD extols the numerous potential health values of NingXia Red Juice, but is not founded on published clinical science.

Nevertheless, although no clinical publications exist on the health benefits of wolfberry juice, there is a growing popular following based sparingly on science and mainly on a large amount of tradition, Chinese lore, appealing taste and effective multilevel marketing.

With the present book, we do not intend to debate these health claims associated with the juice products. In fact, we have a goal to examine the limited scientific information about wolfberry as objectively as possible and to impartially consider health effects inferred from Chinese legends and juice manufacturers. We hope to balance our presentation by using as much information from peer-assessed medical literature as possible.

If some of these health benefits are eventually verified by the appropriate scientific rigors and agreement among experts, then the basic knowledge we hope to provide about wolfberry and its potential use as an ingredient in diets, health-promoting foods and supplements is a worthwhile outcome of this book.

Our main goal is to take a fair view of available information and Chinese lore about this ancient revered plant and help create objective facts to better understand wolfberry's nutrients and phytochemicals. Hopefully, this will provide a good review of the nutrient power wolfberry consumption may contribute toward health.

We shall examine some of the above claims in light of available science. As much of the information on wolfberries comes from Chinese institutions and authors who published only in the Chinese language, western science has had little to advance our understanding to date and has not undertaken many cross-validation studies. Wolfberry has simply not yet caught the imagination of western scientists to undertake a stream of research that would rigorously inspect and test the Chinese data.

Peer-Review for Functional Foods

According to the way in which peer review works, one scientific finding—even if published and accepted by traditionalists years ago in China, should lead to further examination, confirmation, dispute or refute by others. That is how good science is put to the test of scrutiny. One successfully tested idea usually leads to a new one that spawns another, and so on until there is cross-confirmation and general scientific acceptance of given facts.

In 2005, the Institute of Food Technologists published a review by scientific experts of the functional food industry (references, Chapter 12), outlining requirements for establishing credibility of claims about the health benefits of a food or juice such as wolfberry.

Functional foods are those natural or supplemented foods that contain one or more components (nutrients or phytochemicals) imparting a health benefit.

Experts must agree that a "claim is valid based on the totality of publicly available scientific evidence, including evidence from well-designed studies conducted in a manner consistent with generally recognized procedures and principles."

The standard of scientific validity for a health claim includes two components: 1) that the totality of the publicly available evidence supports the substance/disease relationship that is the subject of the claim, and 2) that there is significant scientific agreement among qualified experts that the relationship is valid.

As that chain of proof has not yet been fully established for wolfberry's profile of nutrients and associated health claims, we are reserved about what can be stated.

Therefore, our approach in the book will be to identify available information on wolfberries and present it uninfluenced by commercial motivations.

Value of Clinical Trials

Without belaboring our points above, let's discuss briefly why food and medical research needs the clinical trial system to establish facts about nutrients and health.

Three main factors of a clinical trial that lead to acceptance of facts from nutritional research are 1) that a large number of people, perhaps hundreds or even thousands, have served as subjects, this number representing an even larger population segment (millions of users of the food under study), 2) that the design of the trial, especially its control of dietary or pharmaceutical factors that would influence or disguise the desired result, have been well controlled, and 3) that the results and interpretation of the data have been assessed objectively and reviewed rigorously by other experts ("peers") before publication.

In clinical research on a new drug for treating a medical condition that affects millions of people, these factors are obviously important. Especially the trial design is crucial, but, by nature of the drug being entirely novel to use in people, control of diet or other drugs is relatively easy to establish.

This is not the case in food research where nutrients from many dietary sources can interact and/or conflict with the proposed beneficial nutrients under study. Consequently, it's difficult (perhaps impossible) to establish sufficient experimental conditions for good clinical research on a food source with multiple nutrients affecting health or disease in varied ways.

Some food regulatory authorities, such as the US Food and Drug Administration and the Natural Health Products Directorate of Health Canada, are trying to overcome these problems for clinical trials on food and nutritional products. Chapter 2 references are given in the bibliography, Chapter 12.

Particularly, the Institute of Food Technologists report suggests that a weight of scientific evidence be constructed from 1) epidemiological studies, i.e., large-scale observational data associating foods and disease alleviation, 2) biological mechanisms revealed from chemical, cellular or animal models, and 3) intervention clinical trials of a food on a well-controlled sample of human users.

This preamble about clinical research is provided as background for the upcoming discussions on wolfberry nutrients, especially in Chapters 3-6.

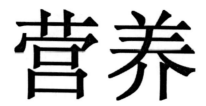

CHAPTER 3
Wolfberry's Nutrient Profile

Nutrient Analysis and Comparisons to Other Superfoods

To put wolfberry's nutrient density into perspective, we gathered information about the concentrations and supposed health benefits of nutrients from other plants reputed as healthy. The objective of this chapter is to show these comparisons and add discussion for how wolfberry stacks up against its competition among so called "superfoods" described by Pratt and Matthews (*SuperFoods Rx*, Chapter 2 references).

In recent years, there has been increasing public attention backed by medical and food science about what nutrients should be included in healthy diets. Intake of nutrient-dense foods and typical servings of them need to be kept in light of *daily recommended intake* levels of nutrients (DRI, related to percent of *daily values, DV*) from government sources such as the US Food and Drug Administration (FDA), US Department of Agriculture (USDA, their RDI data are used in the tables below) and Health Canada who publish dietary guidelines as a service to citizens and food product manufacturers.

The following list is intended to give comparisons between nutrient-rich berries (blueberries vs wolfberries), a fruit (papaya), vegetable (spinach) and grain (flax seed), all recognized as highly nutritious.

Blueberries, spinach and flax seeds, for example, qualify as superfoods in the popular book on nutritious foods by Pratt and Matthews. Our reference data given in the following tables are the most recent values available from several objective sources.

All data for wolfberries were supplied by Rich Nature Nutraceutical Laboratories, Inc., Seattle, either from assays by independent analytical labs contracted by Rich Nature or from Chinese publications translated by this book's coauthors, Dr. Xiaoping Zhang and Richard Zhang.

As an aside relevant to possible future editions of this book, we are interested in other plant candidates included as the world's most nutrient-dense sources and for any documented information on wolfberries we have missed. As an example, a novel "super berry", acai ("ah-sigh-ee", the tropical palmberry), has recently been suggested as the world's most nutritious berry. This attracts our attention to compare with wolfberry so we will present available nutrient data for both berries below and continue to seek information about acai and other nutrient-rich berries.

Accordingly, we invite feedback from readers via email to the address provided on this book's website (copyright page, front of book).

To lay out a foundation for understanding nutrient values in wolfberries, we begin this section by considering nutrient classes in the following way

Macronutrients
- carbohydrates
- fats
- protein
- fiber
- energy (or calories)

Micronutrients
- vitamins
- minerals
- amino acids
- other phytochemicals, such as antioxidants (including pigments like carotenoids), fatty acids, sterols, polysaccharides and others

Particularly due to the interesting high densities and variety of phytochemicals in wolfberries, we give further attention in Chapter 6 to individual novel chemicals making up this category.

We begin our comparisons of wolfberries with other nutritious food sources by considering blueberries, spinach, flax seed, and papaya, each of which at one time has been called by some source "Nature's most nutrient-dense" plant or a highly valued nutritional source for human diets.

Table 1. Macronutrients

Nutrients (per 100 g)	Wolfberry	Recomm Daily Intake	Blueberry	Spinach	Flax Seeds	Papaya
Nutrients (per 100 g)	*Lycium barbarum*	*USDA (adults)*	*Vaccinium angustifolium*	*Spinacia oleracea*	*Linum usitatissimum*	*Carica papaya*
Energy (cal)	370 cal		57 cal	23 cal	492 cal	39 cal
Macronutrients						
Total Fat	8.2 g	**20-35 g**	0.4 g	0 g	34 g	100 mg
Protein	11.7 g	**46-56 g**	0.7 g	3.3 g	19 g	4.3 g
Carbohydrates	67.7 g	**130 g**	14.0 g	3.3 g	34 g	5.9 g
Total dietary fiber	10.0 g	**25-38 g**	2.1 g	3.3 g	27.7 g	1.8 g

The data are presented as available for 100 grams of each source, an amount equal to about 3 ounces or one meal serving. Data for wolfberries are from dried fruit. {Note: if the source data were provided in units different than those presented, we calculated that amount to be equivalent for 100 grams. Data for blueberries, spinach, flax and papaya are from several sources that we compared to choose the most representative numbers. Errors may have occurred in representing the nutrient content of these different sources. We apologize if this is the case and appreciate feedback via the book's website}. The geographic source of wolfberries for the data in this book is the Ningxia Autonomous Region of China (see Chapter 9).

The interesting comparisons in the table give an overall perspective of nutrition provided by the different food sources.

Of particular interest is the carbohydrate content of wolfberries, determined mainly by the high natural sugar and polysaccharide content. Combined with a significant amount of arabinose (table below) and other monosaccharides, polysaccharides are the carbohydrate sources characteristic of wolfberry fruit. Just a 100 gram serving of wolfberries provides about half of the day's needs for carbohydrates, giving a relatively high caloric value (370 calories) justifying wolfberries as an energy food.

Polysaccharides are an excellent source of fermentable "soluble" fiber. Wolfberry's rich content of polysaccharides accounts for its relatively high amount of dietary fiber, with only flax having a higher value among our comparisons.

This is an important health benefit of wolfberries previously not discussed in the scientific literature, so is given a separate chapter (4) in the book.

As we'll also see in greater detail below, the fat in wolfberries comes mainly from the desirable polyunsaturated omega-6 fatty acid, linoleic acid, a "heart-healthy" fat present in its seeds. Blueberries and spinach are mainly fat-free (blueberry seeds are relatively small in numbers and volume, but contain heart-healthy fats), whereas papaya and flax seeds are particularly rich sources of good omega fats. Ground flax seeds especially are renowned among nutritionists for unusually high content of omega-3 fatty acids, mainly from alpha-linolenic acid.

It is interesting that wolfberry's protein content, comparable to that of flax seed—a high-protein grain—is considerably greater than the other fruits shown, blueberries and papaya. Wolfberry fruit is a bounty of amino acids (that collectively make up proteins) and minerals. Horticultural and environmental features are important determinants of inter-specie amino acid and mineral differences among different wolfberry species, as discussed in Chapter 9.

Summarizing the overall macronutrient data for wolfberries, one is impressed by the comprehensive nutrition in a relatively high calorie resource. An excellent fiber source high in protein and total desirable fats, wolfberries are a convenient package for broad-based nutrition compared to other food sources shown. Referenced to the DRI, there is about 30%, 23% and 27% for dietary fiber, protein and fat amounts, respectively, from one serving (100 grams) of wolfberries, representing an excellent supply of macronutrients.

Nutrient by nutrient, wolfberry is most closely comparable in nutritional value to flax seeds, although important differences exist. Among these are wolfberry's "signature" molecules that flax does not contain—polysaccharides and carotenoids—to be discussed in Chapters 4 and 5.

We mentioned the tropical "super"-berry, acai (Euterpe oleracea Mart.), as a nutrient-rich fruit gaining popularity in the United States. It is achieving markets as an ingredient for juices and yogurt smoothies. Acai juice provides 130 calories per 100 gram serving and 150% DV for vitamin C. It has relatively high fiber content (4.5 grams per 100 gram serving, 18% DV) and 4.5 grams of good fats as omega-6 and -9 fatty acids. From these limited data, however, it appears that wolfberries possess a broader spectrum of nutrient density than acai.

Table 2. Fatty Acids

per 100 g of seed oil	Wolfberry Seeds	Recomm Daily Intake, RDI	Blueberry	Spinach	Flax Seeds
	Lycium barbarum	*USDA (adults)*	*Vaccinium angustifolium*	*Spinacia oleracea*	*Linum usitatissimum*
Unsaturated Fatty Acids					
Linoleic	67.8 g	**14-17 g**	0	0	5 g
Alpha-Linolenic	3.4 g	**1.1-1.6 g**	*	0	22 g
Oleic	16.8 g		0	0	7 g
Palmitic	7.3 g		0	0	1.8 g
Stearic	3.2 g		0	0	1.4 g

Data are for fatty acids in seeds. Papaya data were not available.* Alpha-linolenic acid is present in oil of blueberry seeds (Parry et al. 2005, references in Chap. 12)

Omega-3 fatty acids are polyunsaturated, meaning they are multi-unit fat chains containing more than one double bond or monounsaturated having just one double bond, as oleic acid does. They are called omega-3 fatty acids because the first double bond counting from the methyl end of the fatty acid is located at the third carbon atom.

Scientific abbreviations for fatty acids tell the reader something about their structure. The scientific abbreviation for **alpha-linolenic acid** (ALA) is 18:3n-3 (the main omega fatty acid in flax seeds). The first part (18:3) tells the reader that ALA is an 18-carbon fatty acid with three double bonds, while the second part (n-3) tells the reader that ALA is an omega-3 fatty acid attached to the third carbon atom.

ALA is considered an essential fatty acid because it is required for health, but cannot be synthesized in the body so must be eaten. Humans can synthesize other omega-3 fatty acids from ALA, including eicosapentaenoic acid (EPA; 20:5n-3) and docosahexaenoic acid (DHA; 22:6n-3). Because EPA and DHA are abundant in certain species of fish, they are often referred to as marine-derived omega-3 fatty acids, while ALA is considered a plant-derived omega-3 fatty acid. It is this fatty acid that flax seeds offer as a rich source while wolfberry seeds contain modest amounts of ALA—3.4 g per 100 grams.

Linoleic acid (18:2n-6) is another essential polyunsaturated fatty acid that contains 18 carbon atoms, but it differs from ALA in that it is an omega-6 fatty acid and has only two double bonds. This is the major fatty acid found in wolfberry seeds.

Wolfberry seeds contain linoleic acid (67.8 g in 100 ml of seed oil), in an amount equal to about 4 times the DRI, so are a highly enriched source of this valuable fatty acid. Oleic, palmitic and stearic fatty acids are present in wolfberry seeds, indicating a broad-based value for intake of good fats by eating wolfberries, providing the seeds are well-chewed.

In summary, wolfberry, together with acai and seabuckthorn (*Hippophae rhamnoides* L.), another vine berry common to China, provide a comprehensive range of good fat value among berries.

As there are no fats reported for blueberries (except small amounts in seed oil) or spinach, and no data we found for papaya, we focus on a wolfberry vs flax seed comparison in Table 2. Possibly the richest source of good fats among grains, flax seeds provide about 37 grams of polyunsaturated fats in a 100-gram amount, with most of this as ALA.

The ratio of omega-6 to omega-3 fatty acids in the diet of humans eating a well-mixed diet of nutritious foods is probably about 1:1, but the ratio in the typical American diet may be as high as 10:1. This is due to increased use of vegetable oils rich in linoleic acid (omega-6) and declining fish consumption that would provide omega-3 fats. Health scientists suggest that increasing intake of dietary omega-3 fatty acids may provide positive long-term health benefits.

Therefore, eating good plant sources of these fatty acids, as wolfberry seeds offer for linoleic acid and flax seeds for alpha-linolenic acid, provides dietary solutions likely beneficial to human health.

Table 3. Minerals

	Wolfberry	Recomm Daily Intake, RDI	Blueberry	Spinach	Flax Seeds	Papaya
Nutrients (per 100 g)	*Lycium barbarum*	USDA (adults)	*Vaccinium angustifolium*	*Spinacia oleracea*	*Linum usitatissimum*	*Carica papaya*
Minerals						
Calcium	112 mg	**1000 mg**	6 mg	815 mg	197 mg	24 mg
Chromium	30 mcg	**25-35 mg**	-	-	-	-
Copper	2 mg	**900 mcg**	70 mcg	30 mcg	1 mg	0 mcg
Iron	9 mg	**8-18 mg**	0.3 mg	2.7 mg	6.2 mg	71 mcg
Magnesium	109 mg	**320-420 mg**	6 mg	79 mg	362 mg	10 mg
Manganese	1 mg	**2 mg**	0.3 mg	1 mg	3.3 mg	0 mg
Phosphorus	178 mg	**700 mg**	12 mg	49 mg	498 mg	5 mg
Potassium	1132 mg	**4.7 g**	77 mg	556 mg	681 mg	256 mg
Selenium	50 mcg	**55 mcg**	0.07 mcg	1 mcg	5.5 mcg	0.6 mcg
Sodium	150 mg	**1.5 g**	1.0 mg	79 mg	34 mg	3 mg
Zinc	2 mg	**8-11 mg**	0.1 mg	0.7 mg	4.2 mg	71 mcg

Wolfberry data for essential minerals iodine and fluorine were not available. For molybdenum, see below in table for Trace Minerals.

Discussion of minerals

Minerals are inorganic elements from the soil where plants grow and cannot be made by living systems. As plants obtain minerals from the ground and water, most of the minerals in our bodies come directly from plants we eat or indirectly from animal sources consumed as food. Minerals may also be present in the water we drink, but this varies with geographic locale.

Minerals from plant sources also vary from place to place because soil mineral content varies from field to field and region to region. This likely explains different nutrient qualities between similar species of plants growing even in the same province.

Wolfberry is no exception, as its overall edible quality and nutrient content across numerous growing regions in China are known to vary considerably. Berries from Ningxia, for example, are often considered among the Chinese as superior due to richer soil and ideal growing conditions leading to premium quality and taste. We discuss this further in Chapter 9.

In a booklet on goji berries (same as wolfberries, see Chapter 2), Mindell and Handel discuss differences in soil conditions between Ningxia and another prime wolfberry-growing region in China, Xinjiang. They also mention Hebei, Gansu, Qinghai and Shanxi as superior wolfberry growing provinces in China. In common, these regions are traversed by flood plains of the Yellow River or Huang He, the world's most silt-laden river (from which it derives its name due to the yellow muddiness of the water).

From its Himalayan origin at 13,000 ft altitude in western China, Huang He receives runoff from a wide region of mountain slopes and other rivers contributing mineral rich silt as it winds its way from west to east.

Particularly along its way through the Loess Plateau of Gansu Province west of Ningxia, Huang He receives wind-blown erosion that further intensifies the river's silt content. Upon flooding in Ningxia, these factors combine to support concentrated mineral sedimentation that eventually contributes nutrients for wolfberries and all plants growing in downstream regions and flood plains (Chapter 9).

Minerals are inorganic elements used as structural components of cells and as cofactors or catalysts for enzyme activity. Among the body's cells and water compartments, minerals maintain normal osmotic and electrochemical gradients supporting neuromuscular activity and cell membrane functions in animals. Minerals may be required in small amounts (milligrams, mg) or in trace amounts (micrograms, mcg) to serve these physiological functions.

Wolfberry's mineral content is truly impressive, both for the breadth of minerals contained and for their respective densities. For all the minerals shown in the above table, with the exception of chromium, the wolfberry amounts per 100 gram serving are a significant proportion of the RDI.

The amounts per serving for zinc, copper, magnesium, manganese and selenium are a significant percentage of the RDI or, in the case of copper, exceed it by twofold. Indeed, when compared to the plants in our table or any other source, it is rare to find other sources with higher amounts of these 5 minerals, all of which are considered to have properties as cofactors for hundreds of enzymes. The presence in high density of zinc, selenium, copper, magnesium and manganese—each incorporated into numerous enzymes with antioxidant properties—indicates multiple cellular and organ systems in humans that wolfberry minerals may benefit.

As wolfberry's endowment of minerals is so unusually rich, let's briefly cover some medical abstracts providing further definitions of these valuable nutrients.

1. **Publication.** Folia Microbiol (Praha). 2003;48(3):417-26. **Modulatory effects of selenium and zinc on the immune system.** Ferencik M, Ebringer L. Institute of Immunology, Faculty of Medicine, Comenius University, Institute of Neuroimmunology, Slovak Academy of Sciences, Bratislava, Slovakia.

Abstract. Almost all nutrients in the diet play a crucial role in maintaining an "optimal" immune response, and both insufficient and excessive intakes can have negative consequences on the immune status and susceptibility to a variety of pathogens. We summarize the evidence for the importance of two micronutrients, selenium and zinc, and describe the mechanisms through which they affect the immune status and other physiological functions. As a constituent of selenoproteins, selenium is needed for the proper functioning of neutrophils, macrophages, NK cells, T lymphocytes and some other immune mechanisms. Elevated selenium intake may be associated with reduced cancer risk and may alleviate other pathological conditions including oxidative stress and inflammation. Selenium appears to be a key nutrient in counteracting the development of virulence and inhibiting HIV progression to AIDS. It is required for sperm motility and may reduce the risk of miscarriage. Selenium deficiency has been linked to adverse mood states and some findings suggest that selenium deficiency may be a risk factor in cardiovascular diseases. Zinc is required as a catalytic, structural and regulatory ion for enzymes, proteins and transcription factors, and is thus a key trace element in many homeostatic mechanisms of the body, including immune responses. Low zinc ion bioavailability results in limited immunoresistance to infection in aging. Physiological supplementation of zinc for 1-2 months restores immune responses, reduces the incidence of infections and prolongs survival.

Synopsis. Long associated with stimulating immune functions, wolfberry may afford this benefit via its mineral content, particularly for selenium and zinc. This review covered the several immune health benefits provided by these two minerals, including immune cell production, antiviral and anti-infection mechanisms, and general immune homeostasis.

2. **Publication.** Treat Endocrinol. 2004;3(1):41-52. **The role of antioxidant micronutrients in the prevention of diabetic complications.** Bonnefont-Rousselot D. Laboratoire de Biochimie Metabolique et Clinique, Faculte de Pharmacie, Paris, France.

Abstract. Diabetes mellitus is associated with an increased production of reactive oxygen species and a reduction in antioxidant defenses. This leads to oxidative stress, which is partly responsible for diabetic complications. Tight glycemic control is the most effective way of preventing or decreasing these complications. Nevertheless, antioxidant micronutrients can be proposed as adjunctive therapy in patients with diabetes. Indeed, some minerals and vitamins are able to indirectly participate in the reduction of oxidative stress in diabetic patients by improving glycemic control and/or are able to exert antioxidant activity. This article reviews the use of minerals (vanadium, chromium, magnesium, zinc, selenium, copper) and vitamins or cofactors (tocopherol [vitamin E], ascorbic acid [vitamin C], ubidecarenone [ubiquinone; coenzyme Q], nicotinamide, riboflavin, thioctic acid [lipoic acid], flavonoids) in diabetes, with a particular focus on the prevention of diabetic complications. Results show that dietary supplementation with micronutrients may be a complement to classical therapies for preventing and treating diabetic complications. Supplementation is expected to be more effective when a deficiency in these micronutrients exists.

Synopsis. Several micronutrients concentrated in wolfberries, including copper, selenium, zinc, magnesium and vitamin C, are associated in this study with improved outcomes from diabetes mellitus.

Table 4. Vitamins

	Wolfberry	Recomm. Daily Intake, RDI	Blueberry	Spinach	Flax Seeds	Papaya
Nutrients (per 100 g)	Lycium barbarum	USDA (adults)	Vaccinium angustifolium	Spinacia oleracea	Linum usitatissimum	Carica papaya
Vitamins						
Vitamin A*	*	700-900 mcg (approx 666 IU)	54 IU	9367 IU	0 IU	1087 IU
Vitamin B1 (thiamin)	0.153 mg	1.1 mg	7 mcg	100 mcg	200 mcg	0 mg
Vitamin B2 (riboflavin)	1.3 mg	1.2 mg	70 mcg	0.3 mg	0.1 mg	0 mg
Vitamin B3 (niacin)	4.3 mg	15 mg	0.4 mg	0.7 mg	1.4 mg	0.4 mg
Vitamin B6 (pyridoxine)	#	1.3 mg	69 mcg	0.3 mg	0.9 mg	0 mg
Vitamin B12 (cyanocobalamin)	#	2.4 mcg	0 mg	0.1 mg	0 mg	0 mg
Pantothenic acid	#	5 mg	0.1 mg	0 mg	1.5 mg	0.2 mg
Biotin	#	30 mcg	-	-	-	-
Folic acid	#	400 mcg	6 mcg	194 mcg	278 mcg	38 mcg
Vitamin C (ascorbic acid)	29 mg	75-90 mg	9.7 mg	28 mg	1.3 mg	61 mg
Vitamin E	Present in leaves	15 mg	0.6 mg	2 mg	0.3 mg	0.7 mg
Vitamin K	#	90-120 mcg	19 mcg	483 mcg	0 mg	2.6 mg

Vitamin A is converted in the body from provitamin A precursors, such as beta-carotene and beta-cryptoxanthin.Wolfberry contains rich amounts of beta-carotene and beta-cryptoxanthin (Table 6). # no independent reports available.

As substances that must be obtained from dietary sources because they cannot be produced in the body in amounts sufficient to support basic physiological functions essential for life, vitamins are called "essential" nutrients. The term "vitamin" is derived from the Latin word for life "vita", and "amine" because these substances were first thought to consist of amino acids. Vitamins are organic compounds having backbones of carbon, oxygen, and hydrogen, with functional groups containing nitrogen, phosphorus, and other minerals.

Vitamins are considered micronutrients because they are required in relatively small amounts (micrograms or milligrams) when compared to protein, carbohydrate, fat and fiber.

Unfortunately, wolfberry's vitamin contents have not been thoroughly analyzed, with only vitamin C, vitamin B1 (thiamin), B2 (riboflavin) and B3 (niacin) data available. Wolfberry's vitamin C content is considered high (29 mg per 100 g in *dried berries*), similar to spinach, but is only half the level of papaya.

However, in samples of *juice powder concentrate* (requiring 10-11 kg of fresh wolfberries to make one kg of juice powder), the vitamin C content measures 968 mg per 100 g (independent contract assay requested by Rich Nature Nutraceutical Laboratories, Inc., Seattle). We estimate from these numbers that fresh ripe wolfberries contain about 90 mg of vitamin C per 100 g.

Contents for wolfberry riboflavin (vitamin B2) and niacin (vitamin B3) are exceptional. At 1.3 mg per 100 grams, wolfberry riboflavin provides 100% of the recommended day's needs in a single serving. Niacin content is excellent, furnishing 29% of the RDI.

Mono- and polysaccharides

Due to the unusual health benefits attributed to wolfberry polysaccharides, we will devote special attention to these sugar nutrients (Chapter 4) that remain relatively undefined by science and without government advisories on their intake levels. Consequently, there are neither RDI levels nor have there been defined measured amounts of individual polysaccharides in wolfberries—only their presence in the fruit, basic chemical characteristics and in vitro tests on disease models are identified by research to date.

Simpler sugars called monosaccharides have also been found in wolfberries, as shown below.

Table 5. Monosaccharides

	Wolfberry	Blueberry	Spinach	Flax Seeds
Nutrients (per 100 g)	Lycium barbarum	Vaccinium angustifolium	Spinacia oleracea	Linum usitatissimum
Mono-saccharides				
Arabinose	18.8 g	-	-	-
Galactose	6.5 g	-	100 mg	-
Fructose	-	5.0 g	150 mg	-
Glucose	4.7 g	4.9 g	100 mg	210 mg
Sucrose	-	110 mg	70 mg	840 mg
Xylose	900 mg	-	-	-
Mannose	900 mg	-	-	-
Rhamnitol	700 mg	-	-	-

There are no daily reference intake recommendations for monosaccharides. We found no data for papaya.

Discussion of mono- and polysaccharides

Wolfberry research has paid a great deal of attention to polysaccharide properties that remain promising for health benefits to humans. But this research area is young and mainly unfulfilled by scientific standards, providing only identity of these interesting sugar chains and their association with numerous physiological effects, some of them indicating disease prevention.

Among 8 specific polysaccharides identified to date are LBP 1A, 2A and 3A (Lycium barbarum polysaccharide), glycoconjugates LbGp 2, 3, 4 and 5 and Lycium chinense cerebroside. Later in Chapter 4, we develop an understanding of polysaccharides with more background and their potential roles as prebiotic fermentable fibers.

Several monosaccharides have been identified with variable

concentrations in wolfberry fruit as shown above. The contents of arabinose and glucose are exceptional, explaining partly the intense sweetness of wolfberry fruit and its juice. Other contributions toward the sugar content of wolfberries are the monosaccharides, galactose, mannose, xylose and rhamnitol and the previously mentioned polysaccharides.

We present these data as a starting point for further research and comparison with better-understood plants.

Brix

Brix is a measurement system used to express the sugar content (or sweetness intensity) of grapes, wine and related grape juice products, giving a value that can be followed during grape maturity to estimate growth and maturity and harvest timing. Brix values are being used commonly to express the overall sweetness of any fruit and have been assessed now for wolfberry juice, long reputed to be exceptionally sweet at optimum harvest times. A reading of 20-25 Brix is reported as an ideal degree of grape sweetness at harvest for the majority of table wines.

Brix for wolfberry juice has been measured at 26 (courtesy of Department of Food Science, Oregon State University, Corvallis, OR, USA), indicating a sweetness about the same as ripe grapes ready for wine making. Wolfberry's mono- and polysaccharides account for this level of sweetness.

Table 6. Carotenoids

per 100 g	Wolfberry *Lycium barbarum*	Spinach *Spinacia oleracea*	Flax Seeds *Linum usitatissimum*	Papaya *Carica papaya*
Carotenoids				
Alpha-carotene	-	-	-	-
Beta-carotene	7.4 mg	5.6 mg	-	-
Zeaxanthin dipalmitate	161 mg	-	-	-
Free zeaxanthin+	1 mg	-	-	-
Total zeaxanthin	162 mg	12.2 mg	0.6 mg	0.08 mg
Lutein	0.6 mg	7.6 mg	* above	* above
Beta-cryptoxanthin	10 mg	0%	-	-

* *We present data for lutein and zeaxanthin as one value as these carotenoids have nearly identical chemical structure and are usually found together in nature but can be isolated for individual values as done for wolfberries. For the references with *, individual values for lutein and zeaxanthin were not available. There are no daily reference intake recommendations for carotenoids. We found no data for carotenoids in blueberries.*

+ *"Free" zeaxanthin was obtained by saponifying extracts of dried wolfberries. Total zeaxanthin then is the combined amounts of diesterified (dipalmitate) and free components obtained by liquid chromotagraphy and mass spectrometry (courtesy of Prof. DE Breithaupt, Universitat Hohenheim, Stuttgart, Germany, personal communication, 2004 and J Agric Food Chem 51:7044, 2003).*

Carotenoids

Carotenoids are one of nature's most widespread pigments, having received special scientific attention both for their provitamin and antioxidant roles. Nature gives us more than 600 different carotenoids, occurring widely as pigments in plants, microorganisms, and animals.

The most characteristic chemical feature of carotenoids is the long series of double bonds forming the central part of the molecule. This gives them their shape, chemical reactivity, and light-absorbing properties that are clearly such strong characteristics of zeaxanthin and lutein for ocular health (Chapter 5). Beta-carotene, alpha-carotene and beta-cryptoxanthin are provitamin A molecules, converting into vitamin A during metabolism.

Probably the edible plant standard for carotenoid intake is spinach, showing relatively high amounts of beta-carotene and zeaxanthin-lutein. Orange vegetables and fruits, including papaya, carrots, sweet potatoes and pumpkin, are other rich sources of beta-carotene and zeaxanthin-lutein.

Tomatoes, watermelons, pink grapefruits, apricots, and guavas are common sources of lycopene, another carotenoid not presented in Table 6.

Carotenoid pigments have important functions in a plant's photosynthesis and photoprotection. Carotenoids capture and inactivate reactive oxygen species ("oxygen free radicals") such as singlet oxygen formed from exposure to light and air, usually in the fruit's (or the wolfberry's) skin. The same chemical reactions are also associated with its antioxidant activity in human health after eating carotenoid-rich foods like wolfberries.

Zeaxanthin and lutein are excellent lipid-soluble antioxidants that absorb free radicals. There is considerable scientific evidence in human studies to show that carotenoids can prevent lipid oxidation and related oxidative stress.

Because this is an important category of nutrients from wolfberries, we devote a further full discussion of carotenoids and their antioxidant nutritional value in Chapter 5.

This valuable phytonutrient class, for which wolfberries provide high concentrations of beta-carotene and zeaxanthin, still does not have common guidelines for human dietary intakes. The following provides a general guide about dietary carotenoids, from what foods they come and potential health benefits from carotenoid ingestion.

Table 7. Carotenoid food sources and potential health benefits

Carotenoid	Common Food Source	Potential Health Benefit
Alpha-carotene	carrots	antioxidant neutralizing free radicals that may cause damage to cells
Astaxanthin	marine algae, salmon, shrimp	antioxidant
Beta-carotene	wolfberries, various orange or yellow fruits and vegetables	pro-vitamin A antioxidant; contributes to neuronal health and growth
Beta-cryptoxanthin	wolfberries, red peppers	pro-vitamin A antioxidant
Lutein	green, yellow vegetables	healthy vision, neuronal health
Lycopene	tomatoes and tomato products (ketchup, sauces, etc)	may reduce risk of prostate and other cancers
Zeaxanthin	wolfberries, egg yolks, citrus fruits, corn, marigold petals	absorbs blue light, maintains healthy vision; in most sources (wolfberry is an exception), co-distributed equally with lutein

Phenolics

Although wolfberries are well known for having rich carotenoid content—amply supplying antioxidant benefit—the presence of polyphenols in wolfberries may compound their overall antioxidant values. The identical terms "polyphenols" and "phenolic acids" have crept into common language to describe foods like blueberries, red grapes and green tea with exceptional antioxidant value. Because there are many thousands of these complex chemicals found in plants, some of which may yet be confirmed in wolfberries, we shall provide only a brief review and refer to this general phytochemical class as "phenolics".

If substantiated by further science, demonstration of wolfberries having both strong antioxidant classes—carotenoid pigments and phenolics—would be compelling for the overall anrioxidant value of eating this fruit. This would be further evidence supporting the advice of nutritionists—that the consumption of whole foods is best to gain the synergistic benefit of complete nutrition from a single food source like wolfberries.

An interesting question not yet fully explored in food science is whether a food source with more than one class of antioxidants, such as carotenoids combined with phenolics, affords compounded antioxidant protection and health benefits.

Phenolics and their numerous subclasses therefore deserve sufficient attention here just to place this phytonutrient category in perspective among wolfberry nutrients.

Discussion of phenolics

Phenolics generally are categorized as phenolic acids, flavonoids, stilbenes, coumarins, and tannins. Phenolics are the products of normal metabolism in plants, providing essential functions in the reproduction and growth of the plant, acting as defenses against pathogens, parasites, predators and photosynthetic oxygen radicals. They also serve as pigments contributing to colors and astringents (sour tastes) of plants. The deep blue of blueberries and acai, for example, comes from the flavonoid anthocyanins, known to impart antioxidant qualities for these berries. Although not studied sufficiently in wolfberries, there are reports that wolfberries do contain this class of antioxidant pigments.

In addition to their roles in plants, phenolics in the human diet may provide health benefits associated with reduced risk of chronic diseases. It is estimated that flavonoids, of which there are at least 400 types, account for approximately two thirds of phenolics in the American diet.

Flavonoids commonly have a generic structure whose subclass differences classify them as flavonols, flavones, flavanols (catechins), flavanones, anthocyanins, or isoflavonoids.

Flavonols (quercetin, kaempferol, and myricetin), flavones (luteolin and apigenin), flavanols (catechin, epicatechin, epigallocatechin, epicatechin gallate, and epigallocatechin gallate), flavanones (naringenin), anthocyanidins, and isoflavonoids (genistein) are common flavonoids in a diet of colorful fruit and vegetables.

Human intake of all flavonoids is estimated at a few hundred milligrams to 650 mg/day. The total average intake of flavonols (quercetin, myricetin, and kaempferol) and flavones (luteolin and apigenin) was estimated as 23 mg/day of which quercetin contributed about 70%; kaempferol, 17%; myricetin, 6%; luteolin, 4%; and apigenin 3%.

Young Living reports their research on wolfberries shows a high content of the phenolic, ellagic acid, about 26 mg/100 g (References, Chapter 12).

Phytosterols

Just as the animal sterol cholesterol is made naturally in humans, phytosterols ("phyto", from plants) are found in some plants including the wolfberry. The best dietary sources of phytosterols are vegetables, seeds, and nuts. Among berries, beta-sitosterol and daucosterol have been identified in wolfberries, and acai reportedly contains an unnamed sterol(s).

Phytosterols are fat-like plant compounds with chemical structures similar to cholesterol. Over recent years, clinical studies have shown that chronic consumption of phytosterols inhibits absorption of cholesterol by the small intestine and decreases blood levels of low-density lipids (LDL, "bad" fat) and cholesterol by 8-15%. There are no reported serious side effects or adverse reactions to consuming phytosterols. Accordingly, nutritionists are recommending increased dietary intake levels of phytosterols and ingredient manufacturers are creating new phytosterol products as food additives.

When studied for their anti-disease benefits, phytosterols appear to have broad beneficial effects, including stimulation of immune responses often cited as a value of eating wolfberries (Chapters 4,6). Below is an abstract review of health benefits associated with phytosterol consumption.

3. **Publication.** Altern Med Rev. 1999 Jun;4(3):170-7. **Plant sterols and sterolins: a review of their immune-modulating properties.** Bouic PJ, Lamprecht JH. Department of Medical Microbiology, Medical Faculty, University of Stellenbosch. Tygerberg, South Africa.

Abstract. Beta-sitosterol (BSS) and its glycoside (BSSG) are sterol molecules synthesized by plants ("phytosterols"). When humans eat plant foods, phytosterols are ingested and are found in the serum and tissues of healthy individuals, but at concentrations orders of magnitude lower than endogenous cholesterol. Epidemiological studies have correlated a reduced risk of numerous diseases with a diet high in fruits and vegetables, and have concluded that specific molecules, including beta-carotene, vitamin E, vitamin C, and flavonoids, confer some of this protective benefit. However, these epidemiologic studies have not examined the potential effect that phytosterols ingested with fruits and vegetables might have on disease risk reduction. In animals, BSS and BSSG have been shown to exhibit anti-inflammatory, anti-neoplastic, anti-pyretic, and immune-modulating activity. A proprietary BSS:BSSG mixture has demonstrated promising results in a number of studies, including in vitro studies, animal models, and human clinical trials. This phytosterol complex seems to target specific T-helper lymphocytes, the Th1 and Th2 cells, helping normalize their functioning and resulting in improved T-lymphocyte and natural killer cell activity. A dampening effect on overactive antibody responses has also been seen. The re-establishment of immune parameters *may be of help in numerous disease processes relating to chronic immune-mediated abnormalities, including chronic viral infections, tuberculosis, rheumatoid arthritis, allergies, cancer, and auto-immune diseases.*

Table 8. Amino Acids

	Wolfberry	Recomm. Daily Intake, RDI	Blueberry	Spinach	Flax Seeds	Papaya
Nutrients (per 100 g)	*Lycium barbarum*	*USDA (adults)*	*Vaccinium angustifolium*	*Spinacia oleracea*	*Linum usitatissimum*	*Carica papaya*
Amino acids						
Aspartic acid	1951 mg		57 mg	240 mg	9 g	48 mg
Glutamic acid	1882 mg		91 mg	343 mg	1.9 g	33 mg
Proline	1442 mg		28 mg	112 mg	400 mg	10 mg
Arginine	864 mg		37 mg	162 mg	910 mg	10 mg
Threonine*	405 mg	**27 mg***	20 mg	122 mg	420 mg	11 mg
Serine	590 mg		22 mg	104 mg	290 mg	15 mg
Glycine	401 mg		31 mg	134 mg	500 mg	18 mg
Alanine	731 mg		31 mg	142 mg	350 mg	14 mg
Cystine*	196 mg	**25 mg***	8 mg	35 mg	310 mg	-
Valine*	392 mg	**32 mg***	31 mg	161 mg	480 mg	10 mg
Methionine*	92 mg	**25 mg***	12 mg	53 mg	210 mg	2 mg
Leucine*	543 mg	**55 mg***	44 mg	223 mg	570 mg	16 mg
Isoleucine*	319 mg	**25 mg***	23 mg	147 mg	450 mg	8 mg
Tyrosine*	231 mg	**47 mg***	9 mg	108 mg	240 mg	5 mg
Phenylalanine*	316 mg	**47 mg***	26 mg	129 mg	400 mg	9 mg
Lysine	292 mg		13 mg	174 mg	350 mg	25 mg
Histidine*	222 mg	**18 mg***	11 mg	64 mg	250 mg	5 mg
Tryptophan*	137 mg	**7 mg***	3 mg	39 mg	200 mg	8 mg

Sourced only from dietary intake; RDIs not actually established. Asparagine and glutamine data were not available.

Discussion of amino acids

Amino acids are the molecules that make up proteins, the building blocks of cells. All proteins are constructed from some combination of these 20 naturally occurring amino acids.

It is not our intent to go into explanations for each amino acid from wolfberries and how amino acids may contribute to health. For all the amino acids given an RDI, however, wolfberry provides a near-complete source in one serving (Table 8). We do wish to focus on two amino acids—arginine and leucine—that may impart unusual health benefits.

Arginine

Present in wolfberries in a relatively high amount (864 mg per 100 g). L-arginine is a precursor for production of the signaling molecule, nitric oxide, NO (see References to publications by Dr. LJ Ignarro, "Just say NO" and "NO More Heart Disease"). NO is equivalent to the "endothelium-derived relaxing factor", EDRF, a critical hormone controlling the tone of smooth muscle in the vascular system and so is important for blood pressure regulation. NO likely is involved as a signaling transmitter in the functions of all organs.

This is a fascinating area of science that led to thousands of publications in the 1990s and award of the 1998 Nobel Prize in physiology or medicine (LJ Ignarro, above, was co-winner). Understanding NO gives explanation for how drugs such as nitroglycerin and Viagra provide their beneficial effects, and even perhaps how wolfberries have gained their legendary (but clinically unproven) reputation as an aphrodisiac and stimulant of fertility and sexual prowess.

The theory of NO's activity in the cardiovascular system is that NO, a transmitter gas molecule, is synthesized from arginine and acts nearby its site of synthesis. Within milliseconds, it travels over short distances to quickly adjust vascular tone for regulation of blood flow to an organ. The cells lining blood vessels—endothelial cells or endothelium—provide NO as needed, based on a combination of local, blood-borne and neural signals. When NO is made and released, it acts immediately to provide a useful effect, such as a quick relaxation of the vascular smooth muscle controlling increases in blood flow, then is neutralized—all within milliseconds.

There are numerous other ways arginine and NO may affect organ functions, such as through hormonal responses and neural signals. For readers deeply interested, one may search for abstracts on nitric oxide using PubMed (see references in Chapter 12).

Wolfberry has been ascribed with several health benefits that might be explained by this contribution via arginine. From wolfberry consumption, many references to cardiovascular health exist, as do those for priming neuronal activity, increasing energy, sex drive and skin health. All may be related to production of NO from arginine.

Leucine

Leucine is available in the diet from animal protein (poultry, red meats), dairy products, wheat germ and oats. As we show above, leucine content in wolfberries is especially rich, providing more than the RDI from a single serving. Leucine is essential for growth, as it is an element in muscle protein synthesis. Leucine is helpful for healing injuries to skin, muscle, teeth and bones.

Upon metabolism, leucine breakdown produces beta-hydroxy beta-methylbutyrate (HMB), a water-soluble substance that enters a variety of functional pathways possibly influencing the course of protein synthesis and many disorders affected by degeneration of cells and weight control (see References, Chapter 12 for The role of leucine...). HMB may enhance protein metabolism and nitrogen balance in favor of growth by retarding tissue breakdown and encouraging growth of muscle fibers. HMB may stimulate the immune system by enhancing leukocyte (white blood cell) formation, protecting cells from oxidative stress, lowering total and LDL cholesterol, increasing lean body mass and endurance. These effects are all under active research.

As the content of leucine in wolfberries is relatively high and these health characteristics have previously been attributed to eating wolfberries, future research may usefully profit from examining such relationships more thoroughly.

Trace Minerals

For purposes of providing as much information as possible on wolfberries, we list here the trace minerals as determined by independent commercial lab assays contracted by Rich Nature.

Table 9. Trace minerals

Minerals	Content per 100 g
Aluminum	present
Barium	0.01 mg
Boron	2 mg
Lithium	200 mcg
Molybdenum	< 80 mcg
Beryllium	< 30 mcg
Titanium	10 mcg
Strontium	80 mcg
Vanadium	4 mcg
Mercury	< 0.07 ppm
Cadmium	< 50 mcg
Cobalt	< 20 mcg
Chromium	< 0.05 ppm
Nickel	< 3 mcg
Silver	< 0.05 ppm
Tin	20 mcg
Lead	< 0.05 ppm
Arsenic	< 0.10 ppm
Selenium	< 0.05 ppm
Zirconium	< 10 mcg
Niobium	< 10 mcg
Lanthanum	< 20 mcg
Yttrium	20 mcg

Discussion of wolfberry's trace minerals

The definition of "trace" applies to these minerals in microgram amounts (mcg) or parts per million (ppm). Trace minerals likely pertain to good health in diffuse ways, participating mainly as constituents of other molecules or cofactors, but this is a poorly defined area of nutritional science. Some trace minerals are toxic in high concentrations, such as the heavy metals, mercury, lead and silver.

As trace minerals are contained in most foods at appropriate levels, we obtain sufficient intakes through normal diets. There are no regulatory or advisory guidelines for their dietary intakes. We include them here, however, as a reference for future wolfberry research.

Summary: Wolfberry's Main Nutrients

This chapter gathered available nutritional information about wolfberries, indicating that this plant indeed has unusually rich and comprehensive contents of a variety of healthful essential nutrients and phytochemicals. Although several stand out as somewhat unique and rich nutritive constituents, such as the polysaccharides, vitamins C, B2 and B3, several minerals and omega fatty acids in seeds, perhaps the most conspicuous class of phytonutrients collectively are the antioxidant pigment carotenoids to be emphasized in Chapter 5. Nevertheless, all these phytochemicals exist within the wolfberry as one comprehensive package of nutrients, emphasizing further its broad potential benefit as a health food.

This type of nutrient consolidation in one plant has obvious convenience and nutritional value when eaten as a whole food, such as dried wolfberries provide. Taken as a multinutrient food source, wolfberries may furnish health values similar to those associated with antioxidant nutrients, e.g., the two reports below.

4. **Publication.** J Agromedicine. 2003;9(1):65-82. **The antioxidants—vitamin C, vitamin E, selenium, and carotenoids.** Johnson LJ, Meacham SL, Kruskall LJ. Department of Food and Beverage Management, University of Nevada, Las Vegas, USA.

Abstract. This article reviews recent revisions of the Recommended Dietary Allowances (RDA) and the resulting Dietary Reference Intakes (DRI). In April of 2000, the Food and Nutrition Board of the National Academy of Sciences, USA, released Dietary Reference Intakes for vitamin C, vitamin E, selenium, and carotenoids. The central premise of the report did not perpetuate the prevailing popular thought that large doses of antioxidants will prevent chronic diseases. Instead the panel concluded that at this time, insufficient scientific evidence exists to sustain claims that ingesting megadoses of dietary antioxidants can prevent certain chronic illnesses such as cardiovascular disease or cancer.

In some instances recommended nutrient levels were reduced from the previous report in 1989; e.g., for the first time upper tolerable levels of ingestion (UL) were established to prevent the harmful effects of over consumption of essential nutrients, such as vitamin C, vitamin E, and selenium. Although dietary recommendations do exist for vitamin A, the panel did not set recommendations for beta-carotene or the other carotenoids due to lack of sufficient research to support recommended intakes or upper tolerable levels of intake. However, the panel advises the public to avoid intakes of provitamin A compounds, such as the numerous carotenoids, beyond the levels required to prevent vitamin A deficiency. Changes were also made with regard to estimating the amount of provitamin A carotenoids required to make a unit of retinal. The revised estimate suggests a twofold higher conversion rate than previously believed. *Although this comprehensive report on the dietary reference intakes for vitamin C, vitamin E, selenium, and the carotenoids did not decisively confirm the role of antioxidants for the prevention of chronic diseases in humans, many research studies have generated new data to support this concept.*

5. **Publication.** Phytother Res. 2004 Dec;18(12):1008-12. **Antioxidant activities of some common ingredients of traditional Chinese medicine, Angelica sinensis, Lycium barbarum and Poria cocos.** Wu SJ, Ng LT, Lin CC, Graduate Institute of Natural Products, Kaohsiung Medical University, Kaohsiung, Taiwan.

Abstract. The antioxidant activities of three popular ingredients of traditional Chinese medicine, namely Angelica sinensis (AS), Lycium barbarum (LB, wolfberry) and Poria cocos (PC) were evaluated in this study. The results showed that aqueous extracts of these crude drugs exhibited antioxidant activities in a concentration-dependent manner. All extracts displayed an inhibitory effect on FeCl2-ascorbic acid induced lipid peroxidation in rat liver homogenate in vitro, with the order of activity LB > AS > PC. The tested extracts showed a superoxide anion scavenging activity ranging from 28.8% to 82.2% and anti-superoxide activity varying from 38.0% to 84.5%. Among the different extracts, wolfberry extract exhibited the lowest IC50 values (0.77-2.55 microg/mL, i.e., the most sensitivity for effect) in all model systems tested in this study. The present study concludes that wolfberry extract possessed the strongest inhibition on malondialdehyde formation in rat liver homogenate, and superoxide anion scavenging and anti-superoxide formation activities. *These results also suggest that wolfberry extract is a good source of antioxidant agents as a daily dietary supplement.*

Synopsis. This study of a model oxidation system in vitro—homogenized rat liver cells stressed by iron chloride, yielding the marker, malondialdehyde—showed wolfberry extract with the lowest active concentration to inhibit oxidation (most sensitive antioxidant activity) and the strongest antioxidant effect. Effects were compared among other herbal agents used in traditional Chinese medicine, Angelica sinensis (dang gui, a meadow herb) and Poria cocos (a fungus from pine tree roots).

As we review wolfberry's nutritional profile and compare it to those of other high-nutrient foods and the current RDIs, 13 elements stand out with exceptional contents in wolfberries. Where science to date is inadequate to assure their health benefits, we hope further nutritional research will better define their respective roles in a healthy diet.

1. *Polysaccharides, prebiotic fiber*

   As a prebiotic fiber source offering numerous potential health benefits, the wolfberry polysaccharides, perhaps the nutrient most researched in this berry, provide a complex story that remains incompletely developed in science. This nutrient group has such potential importance and interest that we devote special attention to it in Chapter 4.

2. *Vitamin B2 (Riboflavin)*

   An essential vitamin that supports energy metabolism, riboflavin is needed for synthesizing other vitamins and a variety of cofactors affecting enzyme functions. Wolfberry's high concentration of riboflavin, 100% of the RDI from one serving, makes it an ideal food source supporting this essential vitamin and its numerous physiological roles in the body.

3. *Vitamin C*

   Wolfberries are a very rich source of vitamin C, supplying nearly one third of the RDI of this essential vitamin in a single serving. Papaya and spinach are also excellent sources.

   Vitamin C (ascorbic acid) is a water-soluble antioxidant responsible for maintaining iron charges that preserve activity of hundreds of enzymes using iron for metabolism. A principal effect of vitamin C is on collagen fibrils responsible for tensile strength and elasticity in connective tissues like ligaments, tendons and cartilage. Tissues most sensitive to vitamin C status are those containing large amounts of collagen such as blood vessels and capillaries, bone, and scar tissue. Vitamin C affects many body functions including synthesis of brain signaling molecules and production of bile from cholesterol in the liver.

Vitamin C prolongs vitamin E activity so interacts in a positive way to enhance antioxidant capacity in cells.

Daily intake of more than 100 mg vitamin C from a rich food source such as wolfberries may reduce the severity and duration of influenza and colds (see References, Linus Pauling Institute, for excellent discussion).

4. _Beta-carotene_

Long known for its high content of beta-carotene and evident from the deep red color of wolfberries shown on the front and back covers, wolfberries supply an exceptionally rich source of beta-carotene among the comparisons made. Rich Nature contract lab analyses report 7-12 mg per 100 mg serving of wolfberries (depending on harvesting variation, see chapter 10), an extremely rich source of this valuable carotenoid.

A provitamin A carotenoid, beta-carotene is converted in the small intestine to retinol which serves as a precursor for synthesis of vitamin A, then is stored in the body's fat. Some beta-carotene is used as an antioxidant to quench and neutralize oxygen free radicals. Of some 600 carotenoids in nature, most do not participate as precursors of vitamin A.

Vitamin A activity is measured relative to retinal in retinol equivalents. It may be used to support visual functions involving rods and cones of the retina, and is applied in metabolic processes for other tissues.

5. _Zeaxanthin_

Arguably the signature molecule of wolfberries, zeaxanthin content is extremely rich at 162 mg per 100 gram serving, about 13 times higher than spinach.

Possibly wolfberry's most important overall nutrient for human health, zeaxanthin belongs to the carotenoid class so is a member of this valuable antioxidant pigment family. Specifically, however, its role in eye health is a focus for using wolfberries in the diet as a unique, high-density source of zeaxanthin.

With lutein, zeaxanthin is concentrated in the macula lutea region of the eye's retina where the carotenoids appear to have a critical role as pigment filters absorbing blue light that could damage retinal rods and cones—the structural elements called photoreceptors that transmit light into electrical signals for interpreting vision. Consequently, zeaxanthin and lutein are recommended as especially important nutrients by ophthalmologists and eye health support groups for seniors and everyone living in sunny climates.

Due to the importance of zeaxanthin and its unusual concentration in wolfberries, we devote Chapter 5 to emphasize the value of dietary carotenoids to human health.

6. *Copper*

    By relation to RDI as the highest concentration of any mineral in wolfberry fruit, copper is a component of hydroxylase enzymes involved in the synthesis and maintenance of collagen, a base material in the structure of all tissues, especially blood vessels. It is concentrated in muscle, brain and liver, and has high concentration in the smallest blood vessels, capillaries. Consequently, copper can be viewed as an essential cofactor for the body's structure and overall physiological functions.

    Copper also is included as an antioxidant factor, as it participates in the regulation of superoxide dismutase, a critical antioxidant enzyme.

    Wolfberry's generous concentration of copper, at 2 mg per 100 g serving, is twice the RDI but well within tolerable limits for this mineral.

7. *Magnesium*

    Wolfberry magnesium supplies nearly one third of the day's needs in a single serving. Wolfberry is the second highest source of magnesium after flax seeds of the nutrient-dense foods we compared above.

    Magnesium participates in energy metabolism, muscle contraction, nerve impulse transmission, and bone formation. It is required as a cofactor for several hundred enzymes involved in synthesis of fatty acids and proteins.

    Magnesium is important for maintenance of calcium balance at the cell membrane level where the two ions regulate cell activity, particularly for heart and muscle cells. Magnesium and calcium coordinate contractile functions in the smooth muscle cells of blood vessels and so participate in regulation of blood pressure. These two minerals are also essential for bone health.

8. *Potassium*

Wolfberry is an exceptionally good source of potassium, providing over a gram per 100 gram serving. This amounts to about 25% of the daily requirement for potassium and is more than double the amount contributed by other food sources compared.

Potassium is an essential dietary mineral as an "electrolyte" in the body. The term electrolyte refers to a substance that dissociates in solution into charged particles called ions making electrical conduction possible. The normal functioning of our bodies, particularly nerve cell electrical impulses, depends on the exquisite regulation of potassium concentrations both inside and outside cells. High potassium diets are also associated with lower levels of arterial blood pressure.

9. *Selenium*

Wolfberries are an unusually rich source of selenium, containing 50 mcg per 100 gram serving—the day's entire needs—of this important antioxidant cofactor. Wolfberries are by far the richest source of selenium among other food sources compared above.

Selenium is a component of antioxidant enzymes in cell membranes, working together with vitamin E to provide this antioxidant effect. Selenium also has a role in production of hormones, such as prostaglandins important in inflammatory responses and blood pressure control.

10. *Zinc*

Containing 2 mg of zinc per 100 gram serving, wolfberries contribute a high content source of this critical mineral, trailing only flax seeds among the nutritious foods shown in our table. A 2 mg serving of zinc in one wolfberry meal would provide nearly 25% of the day's body needs for this critical mineral, rating it as an excellent source of zinc.

Zinc is a cofactor for over 100 enzymes in the body, especially those involved with the metabolism of protein, carbohydrate, fat and alcohol.

Zinc is essential for protein synthesis, structure and function of cell membranes, tissue growth and repair, wound healing, taste, prostaglandin production, bone construction and fracture healing, blood clotting and neural functions. Considering its role in growth and development, zinc is a crucial mineral for development of children.

11. *Linoleic acid*

Wolfberry seeds are a very rich source of linoleic acid, an omega-6 fatty acid belonging to the "good" fat group—polyunsaturated fatty acids—as are omega-3 fatty acids found in an excellent source like flax seeds. Wolfberry's contribution of linoleic acid from a 100 gram amount of seeds is about one third the RDI.

As mentioned, linoleic and other omega-6 fatty acids belong to the group of "good" fats called polyunsaturated fatty acids. Unlike such "bad" fats as dietary cholesterol and saturated fatty acids (which contribute to heart and other chronic diseases), omega-6s and 3s are beneficial to heart and vascular health. They may also act as a blood thinner by making the blood cells slippery and therefore less likely to stick together.

Omega-6 fatty acids are a type of essential fatty acid people must consume for health, and wolfberry seeds provide a good source of these valuable fats.

12, 13. *Amino Acids, Arginine and Leucine*

Above, we gave evidence that the amino acids, arginine and leucine, found in rich content in wolfberries, have important roles in cellular signaling and growth.

Summary

In this chapter, we provided a review of wolfberry's comprehensive array of phytochemicals and highlighted 13 nutrients concentrated in wolfberries. In the following two chapters, we want to devote closer attention to the wolfberry nutrients with great potential to have disease-specific impacts on nutrition—polysaccharide sugars and the carotenoids.

It is worthwhile summarizing the broader categories of what wolfberry offers as a nutrition source:

Energy. Mainly from its rich source of carbohydrates, wolfberry is a high-energy food.

Macronutrient Synergy. Wolfberry provides good to excellent levels of nutrition from the 4 macronutrient categories—carbohydrates, protein, fats and fiber.

Good Fats. Wolfberry seeds contribute an array of 5 heart-healthy fatty acids, mainly from the omega-6 fat, linoleic acid.

Mineral and Amino Acid Density. Wolfberry's content of every one of 11 essential minerals is exceptional, each falling within the range of "good" to "excellent" amounts according to the USDA guidelines; potassium, magnesium, selenium, zinc and copper are especially high. The 18 amino acids detected in wolfberry fruit provide a high-content source with just one serving for a day's recommended intake.

Vitamins. Although wolfberry's vitamins have not been extensively studied, there is evidence for rich content of vitamins A (from beta-carotene), B2, B3, and C.

Poly- and Monosaccharides. As an intensely sweet fruit with a high brix, wolfberry and its sugar molecules are of special interest for the immune-stimulating and fermentable fiber nutrition provided from poly- and monosaccharides. Despite the sweetness, wolfberry's polysaccharides likely impart a low-glycemic index (low effect on blood sugar) because they are metabolized as fiber rather than degraded to glucose like typical sugars.

Carotenoids. Perhaps the clearest phytochemical signature, wolfberry's rich contents of carotenoid pigments, beta-carotene, beta-cryptoxanthin and zeaxanthin, convey intense antioxidant qualities and so contribute exceptional "pigment power" in a diet containing wolfberries.

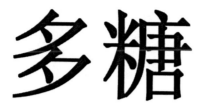

CHAPTER 4
Wolfberry Signature Nutrient: Polysaccharides

Among the various high-density nutrients displayed in the previous chapter are 2 classes worthy to highlight as "signatures" of wolfberry's nutritional character. Each has been the subject of substantial research and inference to significant health benefits of eating wolfberries.

Polysaccharides in wolfberries are chains of sugar molecules that may have direct immune-stimulating properties and are an excellent source of carbohydrate and dietary fiber macronutrition. In this class, we include the monosaccharides presented in Chapter 3.

In the following Chapter 5, we address a second major signature group of wolfberry nutrients, the powerful antioxidant carotenoid pigments, beta-carotene, zeaxanthin ("zee-a-zan-thin") dipalmitate, beta-cryptoxanthin ("krip-toe-zan-thin") and lutein ("loo-teen").

Polysaccharides

Much attention has focused on the nutritional and potential overall health value of wolfberry's polysaccharides (Lycium barbarum polysaccharides or LBPs). Many health benefits of wolfberry consumption are seemingly derived from LBPs but this area of science remains almost totally unconfirmed despite a considerable amount of research done by Chinese investigators.

What are polysaccharides and what evidence in the medical literature exists to support this nutrient class as health promoting?

In this section, we focus on three aspects of wolfberry polysaccharides that eventually may answer these questions.

First, we consider research describing chemical features of wolfberry LBPs. This is limited information but will allow a characterization of what these interesting molecules look like.

Second, apparently for the first time in wolfberry literature, we present the concept that polysaccharides are a source of dietary fiber that imparts numerous potential health benefits. Previous scientists have not addressed the fiber nutrient class as representative of LBPs, but we see the association as an effective broad category that LBPs could contribute to health as fiber sources.

Third, polysaccharides may have direct immune-stimulating properties at the cellular or subcellular level. We will examine related medical literature and provide interpretations where reasonable.

Chemical Identity of Wolfberry Polysaccharides

To begin this section, we present some of the chemical studies obtained from PubMed, the online database of the US National Library of Medicine (Reference in Chapter 2). The structure and function of wolfberry polysaccharides have been described mainly from specific laboratory studies.

As with much of the medical literature on wolfberries, this review is by no means complete due to the relative absence of chemical and biochemical research on wolfberries.

It lacks many of the analyses typical of isolating and defining new phytochemicals, such as structure-activity assays, receptor characterization and binding studies, testing for specificity of action in animal models in vivo, efficacy of various doses of bioactive substances, pharmacological antagonists and other assays required of unknown chemical species to fully define their properties.

Nevertheless, there are a few PubMed citations that allow us to put together a preliminary understanding of wolfberry polysaccharides.

Our format here and throughout the book for reviewing PubMed citations is to provide the "Publication" information, i.e., the journal in which the report appeared, the paper's title and the corresponding date, volume and page location of the publication, authors and their university or industry affiliation. All this information and its format come directly from the PubMed citation.

If an article was written originally only in Chinese, the translators at NIH have noted the paper's Chinese origin by enclosing the title in brackets [like this], indicating that limited information is available and perhaps errors exist in translation to English.

Following that will be the "Abstract" itself. An abstract is a summary of key details describing the research and what was found in the analysis. Often in science journals, the abstract is written to inform other scientists so may be laden with scientific jargon, terms, abbreviations, etc. As we wish to make this information easily understood by non-scientists, we have taken liberties to edit the abstracts and present a review as succinct as possible.

Lastly, in some cases, we offer a synopsis of the research that allows a statement to be made in plain language about why that particular study was important to understanding a property of wolfberries.

1. Publication. Carbohydr Res. 2001 Mar 9;331(1):95-9. **Structural characterization of the glycan part of glycoconjugate LbGp2 from Lycium barbarum L.** Peng X, Tian G. State Key Laboratory of Bio-organic & Natural Products Chemistry, Shanghai Institute of Organic Chemistry, Academia Sinica, People's Republic of China.

Abstract. A glycoconjugate with pronounced immunoactivity, designated as LbGp2, was isolated from the fruit of Lycium barbarum L. and purified to homogeneity by gel-filtration. Its carbohydrate content is up to 90.71% composed of arabinose, galactose and amino acids. The molecular weight is 68.2 kilo-Daltons as determined by size exclusive chromatography. The complete structure of the repeat unit of the glycan of LbGp2 was elucidated based on glycosidic linkage analysis, total acid hydrolysis, partial acid hydrolysis, 1H and 13C NMR spectroscopy. According to the experiments, the glycan possesses a backbone consisting of (1—>6)-beta-galactosyl residues, about fifty percent of which are substituted at C-3 by galactosyl or arabinosyl groups.

Synopsis. This abstract gives a basic chemical characterization of the polysaccharide, LBGp2, a glycan or sugar molecule known by other experiments to have immunoactive properties. It is about 91% sugar, made up mainly of arabinose and galactose units. Weighing 68,200 daltons (a unit of molecular weight) and, by comparison to other macronutrients like proteins (many with molecular weights > 500,000), it is not considered a large molecule.

2. **Publication.** Yao Xue Xue Bao. 2001 Aug;36(8):599-602. [Physico-chemical properties and activity of glycoconjugate LbGp2 from Lycium barbarum L.] [Article in Chinese] Peng XM, Wang ZF, Tian GY. Shanghai Institute of Organic Chemistry, State Key Laboratory of Bio-organic Chemistry, Academia Sinica, Shanghai, China.

Abstract. Aim: To isolate and purify a glycoconjugate (LbGp2) from the fruit of Lycium barbarum L. and study its immunoactivity and antioxidative activity. Methods: By means of gel permeation chromatography, LbGp2 was purified and its physico-chemical properties studied. Results: Molecular weight of LbGp2 was 68,200 daltons and its carbohydrate content was up to 90.7%. Component analysis showed that it was composed of arabinose and galactose in a molar ratio of 3:4, and contained 18 amino acids. The immunologic function and bioactivity of Lbp2 was shown to increase the rate of phagocytosis (cell engulfing), promote lymphocyte translation and accelerate the production of serum hemolysin. LbGp2 had a distinct antioxidant activity against the superoxide anion. Conclusion: LbGp2 was shown to be a glycoconjugate with good immune and antioxidant activities.

Synopsis. By the same researchers as in the first abstract, this study provided evidence that the wolfberry polysaccharide, LbGp2, had phagocytotic activity (could stimulate a cell engulfing process) and could enhance activity of the antioxidant enzyme, superoxide dismutase.

3. **Publication.** Yao Xue Xue Bao. 2001 Mar;36(3):196-9. [Studies on the active polysaccharides from Lycium barbarum L.] [Article in Chinese] Duan CL, Qiao SY, Wang NL, Zhao YM, Qi CH, Yao XS. Affiliation not available.

Abstract. Aim: To investigate the structures and immunomodulation activity of four homogeneous polysaccharides: LBP 1a-1, LBP 1a-2, LBP 3a-1 and LBP 3a-2 isolated from Lycium barbarum L. brought from Zhongning County, Ningxia Province. Methods: Their molecular weights, sugar component (constituents) and their linkages were determined by gel permeation chromatography, acid hydrolysis, periodate oxidation and NMR spectrum. The immunomodulation activity was evaluated with splenocyte proliferation.. Results: Four polysaccharides with molecular weights 115,000, 94,000, 103,000 and 82,000 daltons, were shown to enhance splenocyte proliferation. Conclusion: The four polysaccharides were first isolated from this plant. Polysaccharides made from-polygalacturonans showed stronger immunomodulation.

Synopsis. 4 polysaccharides identified somewhat differently from above as LBP 1a-1, 1a-2, 3a-1 and 3a-2 had immune-stimulating activity as shown by splenocyte proliferation. Their molecular weights varied from 82,000 to 115,000 daltons.

4. **Publication.** Phytother Res. 2000 Sep;14(6):448-51. **LCC, a cerebroside from Lycium chinense, protects primary cultured rat hepatocytes exposed to galactosamine.** Kim SY, Lee EJ, Kim HP, Lee HS, Kim YC. Graduate School of East-West Medical Science, Kyunghee University, Seoul, Korea.

Abstract. Primary cultures of rat hepatocytes (liver cells) exposed to galactosamine (GalN) were used as a screening system to assess whether a new cerebroside, LCC, isolated from the fruits of Lycium chinense, exhibits hepatoprotective activity. Cultured rat hepatocytes injured with GalN routinely release glutamic pyruvic transaminase (GPT) and sorbitol dehydrogenase (SDH) into the culture medium. Treatment of these GalN-injured primary cultures with LCC markedly blocked the release of both GPT and SDH in a dose-dependent manner over several concentrations of LCC ranging from 1 microM to 10 microM. To investigate the mechanism of action for the hepatoprotective activity of LCC, the extent of [(3)H]-uridine incorporation into RNA was measured in GalN-injured cultures of rat hepatocytes. [(3)H]-Uridine incorporation was significantly decreased in injured hepatocytes. LCC, however significantly restored the incorporation of [(3)H]-uridine into RNA in a dose-dependent manner over concentrations ranging from 1 microM to 10 microM. LCC also blocked the suppression of RNA synthesis caused by actinomycin D in a dose-dependent manner. These data suggest that LCC may have prominent hepatoprotective activity and that its therapeutic value should be investigated further.

Synopsis. Using rat liver cells as a model system in vitro, these scientists "injured" the cells by exposing them to galactosamine then tested whether a polysaccharide (a cerebroside) from wolfberries (Lycium chinense, a cultivar of Lycium barbarum) could protect the cells. The wolfberry cerebroside could indeed block the injury in a dose-dependent manner via a mechanism that was mediated through regulation of RNA synthesis.

5. **Publication.** J Nat Prod. 1997 Mar;60(3):274-6. **New antihepatotoxic cerebroside from Lycium chinense fruits.** Kim SY,

Choi YH, Huh H, Kim J, Kim YC, Lee HS. College of Pharmacy, Seoul National University, Korea.

Abstract. Two cerebrosides isolated from Lycium chinense fruits have been characterized. Incubation of hepatocytes with the cerebrosides significantly reduced the levels of glutamic pyruvic transaminase and sorbitol dehydrogenase released by injured cells.

Synopsis. In an earlier study (from 1997) on wolfberry cerebrosides, again using rat liver cells in vitro as the model, the wolfberry polysaccharide extracts protected the cells from chemical toxicity.

6. Publication. Yao Xue Xue Bao. 1998 Jul;33(7):512-6. [Isolation, purification and physico-chemical properties of immunoactive constituents from the fruit of Lycium barbarum L.] [Article in Chinese] Huang L, Lin Y, Tian G, Ji G. Shanghai Institute of Organic Chemistry, Academia Sinica, Shanghai, China.

Abstract. Three glycoconjugates, LbGp3, LbGp4 and LbGp5, were isolated from the fruit of Lycium barbarum L. Molecular weights of LbGp3, LbGp4 and LbGp5 were 92,500, 214,800 and 237,000 daltons, respectively. Carbohydrate contents of LbGp3, LbGP4 and LbGp5 were 93.6%, 85.6%, 8.6%, respectively. LbGp3 was composed of arabinose and galactose in a molar ratio of 1:1. LbGp4 was composed of arabinose, galactose, rhamnitol and glucose in a molar ratio of 1.5:2.5:0.43:0.23. LbGp5 was composed of rhamnitol, arabinose, xylose, galactose, mannose and glucose in a molar ratio of 0.33:0.52:0.42:0.94:0.85:1.

Synopsis. The 3 wolfberry polysaccharides, LbGp3, 4 and 5, were characterized for molecular weight and sugar composition. LbGp3 was found to be a 92,500 dalton conjugate, whereas LbGp 4 and 5 were 215,000 and 23,700 daltons, respectively. The rank order for total sugar content was 94%, 86% and 9%, respectively, for LbGp3, 4 and 5. In other words, the sugar contents of LbGp 3 and 4 are about 10x the sugar content of LbGp5. From analysis of the individual monosaccharides, it appears that the more arabinose and galactose in the molecule, the higher its sugar content.

7. Publication. Wei Sheng Yan Jiu. 2000 Mar 30;29(2):115-7. [Isolation and purification of Lycium barbarum polysaccharides and its antifatigue effect] [Article in Chinese] Luo Q, Yan J, Zhang S. Department of Hygiene, Hubei Medical University, Wuhan, China.

Abstract. A purified component of lycium barbarum polysaccharide

(LBP) was isolated from lycium barbarum L. by gel chromatography. LBP was tested on five different doses (5, 10, 20, 50 and 100 mg.kg-1.d-1) in mice. The results showed that LBP induced a remarkable adaptability to exercise load, enhanced resistance and accelerated elimination of fatigue. LBP could enhance the storage of muscle and liver glycogen, increase the activity of enzymes neutralizing lactic acid before and after swimming, decrease the increase of blood urea nitrogen after strenuous exercise, and accelerate the clearance of blood urea nitrogen after exercise.

Synopsis. All the effects observed in this study are signs of improved tolerance to exercise and fatigue due to a wolfberry polysaccharide given to mice.

Summary: from the above 7 chemical studies, wolfberry polysaccharides have chemical characteristics that vary from one to another, including their molecular weight and, by inference, their molecular diameter (size), a measure critical to permeation across cell membranes in biological systems. Overall number of sugar units, prevalence of one monosaccharide vs another (and corresponding effect on "brix" or sweetness), order of the sugar chains, types of links between units, branch points in the molecule's backbone and whether acidic groups are attached were other characteristics defined.

This variety of molecular design has potential physiological and pharmacological significance for individual polysaccharides, as future studies on receptor binding, dose-response relationships and antagonist identification will hopefully reveal.

Polysaccharides: Focus on Fermentable Fiber

Consumed as long as people have eaten plants, dietary fiber has recently entered into view of government, nutrition advisory groups and the public as one of our most important dietary macronutrients.

Chronic intake of fiber through foods like fresh fruit, vegetables, whole grains and nuts is now associated with reduced risk of some of the world's most prevalent diseases, such as obesity, diabetes, high blood cholesterol, cardiovascular disease, and numerous gastrointestinal disorders. In this last category are constipation, inflammatory bowel disease, ulcerative colitis, Crohn's disease, diverticulitis and colon cancer—all disorders of the intestinal tract where fiber can provide healthful benefits.

Recent medical research has proven several beneficial effects of consuming fiber, among which are improved absorption of calcium, magnesium, and iron, reduction of blood cholesterol, stabilization of blood glucose levels, maintenance of the intestinal environment and stimulation of immune responses.

Recognizing these facts, advisories now exist in several countries for increasing intake of dietary fiber to approximately 30 grams per day, up by 200% from current intake levels. But achieving this goal has been difficult because high-fiber foods do not always taste good or lack other properties sufficiently appealing to attract them into regular dietary practices. Consequently, less than half of American adults and even a lower percentage of children consume the recommended level of fiber.

Defining Fiber and Polysaccharides

Over the past 30 years, government agencies around the world including the US FDA have undertaken analyses and definitions of fiber to more accurately describe this dietary nutrient. Among some 32 reports filed, the most universally accepted seems to be one in 2000 by the American Association of Cereal Chemists. This AACC group focused on the physiological and metabolic significance of fiber.

The AACC defined dietary fiber as *"the edible parts of plants or similar carbohydrates resistant to digestion and absorption in the human small intestine with complete or partial fermentation in the large intestine"*.

Let's review—digestion-absorption-fermentation of a food source called "resistant starch" refers to fiber sources resistant to complete digestion, so they may pass through our system perhaps only attracting water along the way. We should remember these terms because they are normal healthy physiological processes that influence how fiber works in the body and what benefits it provides.

"Fermentation" is one normal biological process many people never consider when they eat healthy foods like fresh fruits or vegetables. Fermentation simply is the breakdown of carbohydrate (sugar) molecules in the large intestine, yielding gases and further useful chemicals like short-chain fatty acids. Arguably, fermentation is the primary digestive fate for wolfberry polysaccharides.

Dietary fiber sources include polysaccharides (starch or sugar chains of dozens to many hundreds or thousands of units), oligosaccharides (short-chain sugars, usually 2-20 units long), monosaccharides, lignins and even "insoluble" fiber sources like cellulose. In all plants, both soluble and insoluble fibers coexist in variable proportions.

Examples of polysaccharides mentioned in public literature on dietary fiber include

- pectins, a seed-like component common in fruits, berries, legumes
- cellulose from brans, beets, many vegetables
- beta-glucans in oats
- plant waxes from many edible species
- polyfructoses from inulin and oligofructans
- gums and mucillages from tree exudates (gum acacia), algae (agar, carageenan) and grain seeds (psyllium seed husk)

Fermentation of Polysaccharides and Prebiotic Nutrient Value

The process of intestinal fermentation involves action by natural bacteria, sometimes called flora, residing in our large intestine (primarily the colon) and how those bacteria use soluble fiber sources in the process of fermentation to produce valuable chemicals and health benefits.

Since the fiber serves as food for the bacteria, this is called a "prebiotic" nutrient value, meaning that before the bacteria can serve their main purpose in digestion—producing enzymes that digest food—they must be fed with a substrate they prefer, i.e., fermentable fibers.

Wolfberry polysaccharide soluble fibers can provide this prebiotic function in the fermentation process.

Fermentation is a metabolic activity involving use of one organic source to create others, such as by using enzymes to digest food then releasing new elements (e.g., nutrients) for absorption into the circulating blood and body fluids. Among products of fermentation are gases (methane, carbon dioxide, hydrogen, nitrogen) and short-chain fatty acids as new molecules clipped from the more complex digested fiber and food compounds.

Fatty acids such as butyric acid, acetic acid, propionic acid and valeric acid have several beneficial physiological effects in the large intestine deserving our closer attention below. These fatty acids make up about 90% of the total fatty acid yield from fermentation in the human body.

Insoluble fiber sources from plants, such as cellulose, typically undergo little fermentation so do not contribute new elements that may affect health. They do, however, bind water effectively so are valuable in digestion as stool softening agents with clear benefit promoting laxation and regularity.

For perspective, "probiotic" nutrients are those that add already-active bacteria to the intestinal tract from the diet. Included here are yogurts with live bacterial cultures and some fermented cheeses or milk products. Dietary fiber in the form of wolfberry constituents does not contribute probiotic value in foods as the bacterial cultures must be live.

Wolfberry Polysaccharides as Fermentable Fiber or Resistant Starch

Introduced with this book is a new concept for defining wolfberry polysaccharides as soluble or fermentable fiber sources, also called resistant starch by some scientists. The polysaccharides or starch molecules are not really digested per se, but rather enter more subtle forms of intestinal metabolism such as fermentation or absorption of water to create a gel mass.

Given this definition, an interpretation about the potential health benefits of wolfberries is gained from how other plant's polysaccharides may contribute health benefits to humans.

For example, beta-glucans (present in oats and Ganoderma mushrooms, see abstract #8 below in this chapter) are polysaccharides that can modulate cell-mediated immune responses.

These agents are known as "biological response modifiers". They appear to act by binding to specific receptors on T-cells and macrophages (cells involved in immune functions), causing cellular responses that include the production and release of immune-promoting cytokines such as tumor necrosis factor (TNF) and interleukins. Cytokines are messenger molecules that regulate immune and inflammatory processes. The presence of these receptors on immune cells provides protection against many bacteria and fungi that contain beta-glucans and similar polysaccharides in their cell walls. Accordingly, this is one mechanism for how oats and mushrooms provide their well-known health benefits.

Our focus is on the digestion of wolfberries in the large intestine, the most heavily colonized area of the digestive system containing over a billion bacteria for every pea-sized amount of food entering the large intestine.

As the food mass containing wolfberry polysaccharides undergoes fermentation, polysaccharides contribute a prebiotic value to the flora (bacteria) whose end-products include several short-chain fatty acids positively linked to a variety of health benefits.

Given the overall health importance of these fatty acids, we devote the separate section below to their possible actions.

Production of Short-Chain Fatty Acids

Available science supports our hypothesis that wolfberry polysaccharides undergo normal fermentation. This information allows us to postulate that all or some of their benefit as a fiber source is fermented to valuable short-chain fatty acids.

When produced by fermentation in the colon, short-chain fatty acids—primarily butyric acid, acetic acid and propionic acid—can increase absorption of minerals (calcium, iron, magnesium), inhibit growth of pathogens on the intestinal wall by increasing the acidic content (in science, this is called a decreased pH) of the lower large intestine—the colon—and by providing energy substances as food for the mucosal layers of the intestine.

It is likely that an increased acidic environment in the colon promotes solubility of minerals and so enhances their availability for absorption. It has also been speculated that increased acidity inhibits growth of colonic and rectal tumors.

Should these fatty acids be transported into intestinal venous blood or absorbed via lymph channels, they reach the systemic circulation and can be deposited in the liver and kidneys where they have useful roles in the functions of those organs. From studies done on isolated liver cells or liver enzymes, for example, some Chinese authors have speculated that wolfberry consumption has a specific benefit for liver health.

Fatty acids also inhibit cholesterol synthesis and lipid deposition, stabilize circulating glucose levels (helpful in management of diabetes and weight control) and reduce uric acid levels (and so may relieve gout). All these factors promote health of the cardiovascular and skeletal systems.

Health-Related Implications for Polysaccharide Fermentation

Colon and Rectal Cancers

Among the most severe and morbid cancers in North America and Europe, colon cancer has been the object of epidemiological studies finding that increased consumption of high-fiber foods such as fresh vegetables and fruits can be preventive against this disease.

Specifically, the European Prospective Investigation on Cancer, a major multinational clinical trial involving half a million people, found that dietary fiber provides colonic and rectal protection from formation of cancerous polyps.

Interpreted from this study was that polysaccharides, acting as prebiotics for colonic fermentation, increased the number and kinds of bacteria and changes in bacterial metabolism that included activity against toxins, carcinogens and tumor promoting cells.

Therefore, several mechanisms of anti-tumor activity may be stimulated in the large intestine by consumption of wolfberries or any food source rich in polysaccharides.

Apoptosis

A relatively new term in modern scientific literature (since the 1970s), apoptosis ("eh-poe-toe-sis") refers to the natural dying process of all cells, including unwanted cells like those at the origin of cancers. Stimulating apoptosis specifically of cancer cells, for example, would be desirable, perhaps causing them to die faster before becoming metastatic.

One of the intriguing current theories of the beneficial effects of fermentable fiber in cancer is that short-chain fatty acids formed during fermentation, especially butyric acid, reduce the pH (raise acidity levels) in the large intestine, stimulating apoptosis of cancer polyps. This means that cancer cells may die faster than they would under neutral or high pH conditions that result from low-fiber diets.

Other possible effects of wolfberry polysaccharide fermentation in the colon include stimulation of bile acid secretion (which would also decrease pH or increase acidity), increased absorption or metabolism of substrates needed by cancer cells, speeding the transit time of the colonic contents (so reducing the time for uptake of nutrients by cancer cells) and/or direct inhibition of cancer polyp metabolism by the short-chain fatty acids produced during polysaccharide fermentation.

These mechanisms need to be confirmed by additional research but offer a reasonable set of hypothetical conditions supporting addition of fermentable fibers to one's diet to enhance immune defenses against cancer.

Rich in polysaccharides, wolfberries would be one of many easy-to-use natural food sources for gaining this promising health protection.

Diabetes

Following a meal, the normal response in humans is to secrete the pancreatic hormone, insulin, into the circulation to promote food-derived glucose (sugar) being used as fuel or deposited in body tissues. In diabetics, this response is frustrated by inability of the pancreas to secrete insulin in proper amounts or at all, allowing blood sugar levels to rise rapidly for sustained periods. Glucose remains in the blood rather than being transported into tissues for storage or use by cells.

With so much of a circulating sugar burden, the kidneys produce more sugar-laden urine in a futile attempt to restore normality, leaving the person thirsty, hungry, emaciated, weak and possibly disoriented with a very high sugar level in the blood and low level in tissues demanding fuel. The brain is especially insistent for glucose, so disorientation follows readily in a diabetic patient untreated by insulin injection.

With glucose unavailable in the body's tissues, the diabetic relies on fat and protein metabolism for energy, leading to labored breathing, high fat levels in the blood, circulatory difficulties especially in the extremities, production of ketones that give the breath a metallic smell and reduced resistance to infections.

Over the past 35 years, there has been accumulating evidence that dietary fiber can reduce the risk for developing diabetes mellitus. Particularly food sources with fermentable polysaccharides offer the greatest possible benefit for decreasing the glycemic response to a meal and for increasing one's sensitivity to insulin.

How fermentable fibers do this remains scientifically undefined but probably involves again those short-chain fatty acids—butyric, propionic and acetic acid that together may help regulate uptake of sugar and other nutrients into tissues. Another factor may result from the viscous and gelatinous nature of fiber-rich contents in the intestine, reducing transit time and enhancing mineral absorption in ways that assist the handling of sugars by our cells.

Lipid Metabolism and Cardiovascular Disease

Likely the first and most widely recognized benefit of dietary fiber is for reducing risk of lipid-associated cardiovascular diseases. Markers of such disorders—circulating levels of cholesterol and low-density lipoprotein (LDL)—are diminished by long-term dietary intake of fermentable polysaccharides.

The well-known fermentable fiber source, psyllium seed husk powder (Plantago ovata, e.g., Metamucil), has been allowed an FDA claim stating that chronic ingestion of psyllium can reduce cholesterol levels and lower the risk of heart disease.

Although there are numerous possible explanations for this effect, the most compelling scientific evidence is that the short-chain fatty acids produced by polysaccharide fermentation inhibit formation of other fatty acids, decrease gene expression for synthesis of new lipids, and depress the production of triglycerides. Overall, circulating amounts of lipids are reduced by diets containing fermentable fibers.

Interestingly, these same effects are at the basis for lowering arterial blood pressure (relieving hypertension) and curbing appetite, and so protect against weight gain.

Bone Health

Calcium is the most common mineral in the human body, about 99% of it being located in bones and teeth, while the rest is found in blood and soft tissues. Calcium levels in blood and fluid surrounding the cells (extracellular fluid) must be maintained within narrow limits for normal cell functioning. Calcium is so vital to survival that the body will demineralize bone to maintain normal blood calcium levels when calcium intake is insufficient.

A cofactor in how calcium is used in cells, magnesium plays important roles in structure and function of the body's organs. The adult human body contains about 25 grams of magnesium, over 60% of which is found in bones.

Transport of calcium, magnesium and iron across the wall of the small intestine is stimulated by the short-chain fatty acids as products of polysaccharide fermentation.

Some studies have shown that this same effect occurs in the colon, providing a more distal opportunity during digestion for nutrient uptake, even late in the passage of food and stool contents through the intestinal tract.

Intestinal System

As mentioned above, the billions of "good" bacteria in the intestine are involved not only in the several stages of digestion, nutrient absorption and waste elimination but also for general health of the intestinal wall and its many functions. The intestinal system is a major immune organ, functioning as a barrier to toxins that might otherwise gain access to the systemic blood or be absorbed with water into the lymph system.

The integrity of this barrier can change with a variety of illnesses associated with translocation of bacteria, such as enteritis (small intestine inflammation), Crohn's disease (inflammation specifically of the small intestinal ileum), colitis, diverticulitis, ulcers, adverse reactions to antibiotics, and parasitic infections.

The end products of fermentation of polysaccharides—including again those short-chain fatty acids—create physiological conditions that promote growth of healthy bacteria and minimize formation of pathogens. Particularly butyric acid regulates apoptosis and cell division while providing intestinal epithelial cells a source of energy.

Lessons about Wolfberry Polysaccharides from Ganoderma lucidum (Reishi mushrooms)

To gain insights about how wolfberry polysaccharides may contribute to healthful effects, let's have a look at a plant more extensively studied for its herbal medicinal values—Ganoderma mushrooms, another native herb of China and long included among traditional Chinese remedies.

8. Publication. Mini Rev Med Chem. 2004 Oct;4(8):873-9. **Cellular and physiological effects of Ganoderma lucidum (Reishi).** Sliva D. Methodist Research Institute, Clarian Health Partners, Inc., Indianapolis, IN, USA.

Abstract. In Asia, a variety of dietary products have been used for centuries as popular remedies to prevent or treat different diseases. A large number of herbs and extracts from medicinal mushrooms are used for the treatment of diseases. Mushrooms such as Ganoderma lucidum (Reishi), Lentinus edodes (Shiitake), Grifola frondosa (Maitake), Hericium erinaceum (Yamabushitake), and Inonotus obliquus (Chaga) have been collected and consumed in China, Korea, and Japan for centuries. Until recently, these mushrooms were largely unknown in the West and were considered 'fungi' without any nutritional value. However, most mushrooms are rich in vitamins, fiber, and amino acids and low in fat, cholesterol, and calories. These mushrooms contain a large variety of biologically active *polysaccharides with immunostimulatory properties,* which contribute to their anticancer effects. Furthermore, other bioactive substances, including triterpenes, proteins, lipids, cerebrosides, and phenols, have been identified and characterized in medicinal mushrooms. This review summarizes the biological effects of Ganoderma lucidum upon specific signaling molecules and pathways, which are responsible for its therapeutic effects.

Synopsis. As with wolfberries, edible Ganoderma (or Reishi) mushrooms are packed with nutrients that seemingly have a broad array of health benefits. Considerably more medical literature is available on Ganoderma mushrooms than on wolfberries.

Consequently, there are lessons to be borrowed about how wolfberry nutrients may behave similarly to those in Ganoderma mushrooms. Our assessment of Ganoderma will not be extensive but rather focused to this one review article, Ganoderma nutrients and potential health benefits applying to both plants.

Ganoderma lucidum has been a staple of Chinese traditional medicine for about the same length of time as wolfberries—thousands of years. Ganoderma has been recorded in Chinese materia medica as beneficial for longevity, general vitality, and prevention or relief from a number of diseases affected by immune dysfunction, such as allergies and perhaps cancer.

These health benefits appear to stem mainly from two nutrient groups—polysaccharides and triterpenes. We shall cover each separately as it relates to similar wolfberry components.

Ganoderma Polysaccharides

Much of the attention for Ganoderma applications in traditional Chinese medicine has focused on the mushroom polysaccharide ability to inhibit tumor development and progress of cancer. More than 100 different polysaccharides have been isolated from Ganoderma lucidum, the most active of which are in the form of beta-D-glucans. The polysaccharide effect may be mediated through a cell receptor that binds with the beta-glucan polysaccharides that involve

- inhibiting the growth and cell-division process of leukemia cells
- inducing apoptosis of cancer cells
- stimulating interleukin production, inhibiting tumor activity
- stimulating phagocytosis that engulfs tumor cells and neutralizes them
- creating an antioxidant effect that absorbs and neutralizes radical oxygen species
- inhibiting viral species, such as herpes simplex
- inhibiting enzymes called polymerases needed for cells to replicate and so may stop cancer cells from forming and metastasizing (spreading randomly via the blood throughout the body)

As such studies have not been done to date for wolfberry, we can only speculate about whether wolfberry polysaccharides provide similar benefits, but the information for mushroom polysaccharides gives valuable insights about such immune-enhancing properties and their mechanisms of action.

Ganoderma Terpenes

Terpenes (and triterpenes) are a class of dozens of hydrocarbon-containing chemicals (including carotenes from wolfberries) found in species like the edible Reishi mushroom, Ganoderma lucidum.

A comparison of terpenes from mushrooms or wolfberries leads us to consider the carotene class, a group of orange pigments important for photosynthesis. Carotenes are responsible for the orange color of plants like carrot, tomato and wolfberry, transmitting the light energy it absorbs to chlorophyll.

Carotene comes in two forms—alpha and beta-carotene, a major component of wolfberries. As a general rule, the greater the intensity of orange color in a fruit or vegetable, the more beta-carotene it contains.

We discuss this terpene significance here for the background on Ganoderma mushrooms (whose terpenes are not likely carotenes), but a more detailed review of carotenes and other carotenoids specifically found in wolfberries is given in the next chapter.

Numerous biological effects with potential health benefits are associated with Ganoderma terpenes

- toxic against liver, lung, breast, muscle (sarcoma) and nose/throat cancer cells
- prevent circulating cancer cells from binding in new organ locations
- induce apoptosis of breast cancer cells
- inhibit enzymes involved in replication of the HIV-AIDS virus
- inhibit blood platelet response to thromboxane-A, meaning that blood clotting mechanisms would be inhibited

The above results were obtained mainly by isolation of a polysaccharide or terpene from Ganoderma mushrooms then testing it on a specific cell type or organ, usually in vitro.

In life, eating the whole mushroom (or wolfberry) would likely achieve cumulative biological or medicinal effects greater than those of an individual nutrient—this is the rationale behind the theory of *phytonutrient synergy* explained in Chapter 2, i.e., multiple nutrients from whole food interacting synergistically and beneficially.

As with polysaccharides, however, we do not have sufficient information to determine whether wolfberry terpenes exist in quantities active for health benefits or what their properties actually are. The above effects, however, are interesting and provide a basis for further study on this class of nutrients.

As a related note, wolfberry carotenoids, particularly beta-carotene (Chapter 5), may fulfill the chemical requirements for providing the terpene benefits discussed above. Carotenoids are sometimes referred to as "terpenoids".

Mindell and Handel: Polysaccharides as Wolfberry "Master" Molecules

In their book, "Goji—The Himalayan Health Secret" (2003), Mindell and Handel discuss the polysaccharides from wolfberry as "master molecules by virtue of their ability to command and control many of the body's most important biochemical defense mechanisms."

They list the following as health benefits from goji (wolfberry) polysaccharides, each being consistent with preliminary science presented as abstracts in this chapter

1. inhibit tumor growth
2. prevent cancer
3. neutralize side effects of chemotherapy and radiation
4. help normalize blood sugar
5. combat autoimmune disease
6. act as an anti-inflammatory
7. balance immune function
8. lower cholesterol and blood sugar
9. increase calcium absorption

The authors provide an interesting but untested hypothesis that wolfberries manufacture polysaccharides as defense molecules for their own protection against environmental extremes of seasonal temperatures, high altitude, variable precipitation, parasites, fungi, etc. By eating wolfberries, humans would gain these same defenses.

The Mindell-Handel book presents analyses by spectrometric fingerprinting of wolfberries from different regions of China, with the autonomous regions of Xinjiang and Ningxia having the highest peaks indicating the presence of greater amounts of polysaccharides from these two regions. The authors conclude that more high spectral peaks correlate positively with a higher density of bioactive polysaccharides and so impart greater health potency of such wolfberries.

As these findings appear unconfirmed by science in peer-reviewed medical literature, we feel it is premature to regard the conclusions as fact. However, we can comment that such relationships are not definitive proof of spectral peaks representing *only* polysaccharides with biological potency. For one example among several possibilities, other unidentified phytochemicals could be represented in those peaks.

Mindell and Handel also use the information to explain why wolfberries from Xinjiang and the Hunza Valley of the Himalaya Mountains (having the highest spectral peaks) are, in their view, the premium berries known inside and outside China. This information also has not received objective assessment. By other sources, berries from Chinese regions like Ningxia also make that claim.

This discussion leads to geographic and environmental factors affecting wolfberry farming and perhaps the quality of wolfberries from different geographic regions of China, a topic discussed further by Mindell and Handel and one we cover in Chapter 9.

Wolfberry Polysaccharides—Medical Literature

Most of the science on wolfberries has been done in China and other southeast Asian countries where the fruit's respected reputation for health and healing has lived for thousands of years.

In the West, we have limited ability to judge this science sufficiently. The published work is usually in Chinese and our access to English translations of the full medical literature on wolfberries comes only from the ability of scientific translators to provide accurate summaries of the full publications.

Polysaccharides: Miscellaneous Citations from PubMed

9. Publication. Wei Sheng Yan Jiu. 2003 Nov;32(6):599-601. **Study on protective action of lycium barbarum polysaccharides on DNA impairments of testicle cells in mice** [Article in Chinese] Huang X, Yang M, Wu X, Yan J. School of Public Health, Wuhan University, Wuhan, China.

Abstract. To investigate the protective effect of lycium barbarum polysaccharides (LBP) on DNA oxidative damage of testicle cells induced by hydrogen peroxide (H2O2). The single cell gel electrophoresis was used to detect the breakage of DNA strand and analyze LBP protection against oxidation damage in testicle cells treated by different concentrations of LBP for 1 hour firstly, and then cultured with 100 mumol/L H2O2 for 25 min. The results showed that H2O2 could induce the breakage of DNA strand. Pretreatment with LBP (50, 100, 200, 400 micrograms/ml) significantly decreased the frequencies of damaged cells treated by H2O2. LBP itself could absorb the free radicals and restrain the DNA damage of testicle cells caused by oxidative stress.

Synopsis. Using testicular cells as an in vitro model, these authors showed that LBPs protected DNA in the cells against oxidative damage by hydrogen peroxide.

10. Publication. Yao Xue Xue Bao. 2001 Feb;36(2):108-11. **[Studies on the glycoconjugates and glycans from Lycium barbarum L in inhibiting low-density lipoprotein (LDL) peroxidation]** [Article in Chinese] Huang LJ, Tian GY, Wang ZF, Dong JB, Wu MP. State Key Laboratory of Bio-organic and Natural Products Chemistry, Shanghai Institute of Organic Chemistry, Chinese Academy of Sciences, Shanghai, China.

Abstract. Aim: To determine the effects of glycoconjugates and their glycans from Lycium barbarum L. on inhibiting low-density lipoprotein (LDL) peroxidation. Methods: Using copper-induced oxidation as a model, the oxidative production of thiobarbituric acid-reactive substances was measured. Results: The effects of glycoconjugates and their glycans from Lycium barbarum L. on inhibiting LDL peroxidation were different, among them, glycoconjugate LbGp5 showed the best effect on inhibiting LDL peroxidation. Conclusion: The glycoconjugates can inhibit LDL peroxidation while their glycans showed no effects on inhibiting LDL peroxidation.

Synopsis. Polysaccharide LbGp5 showed strong antioxidant activity for inhibiting low-density lipoprotein peroxidation whereas the glycan components did not have antioxidant activity.

Health and Disease Properties

Cancer

11. **Publication.** Zhonghua Zhong Liu Za Zhi. 1994 Nov;16(6):428-31. **[Observation of the effects of LAK/IL-2 therapy combining with Lycium barbarum polysaccharides in the treatment of 75 cancer patients]** [Article in Chinese] Cao GW, Yang WG, Du P. Second Military Medical University, Department of Microbiology, Shanghai, China.

Abstract. Seventy nine advanced cancer patients in a clinical trial were treated with lymphokine-activated killer cells (LAK)/interleukin-2 combining with Lycium Barbarum polysaccharides (LBP). Initial results of the treatment from 75 evaluable patients indicated that objective regression of cancer was achieved in patients with malignant melanoma, renal cell carcinoma, colorectal carcinoma, lung cancer, nasopharyngeal carcinoma,_malignant hydrothorax. The response rate of patients treated with LAK/IL-2 plus LBP was 40.9% while that of patients treated with LAK/IL-2 alone was 16.1% (P < 0.05). The mean remission in patients treated with LAK/IL-2 plus LBP also lasted significantly longer. LAK/IL-2 plus LBP treatment led to more marked increase in NK and LAK cell activity than LAK/IL-2 without LBP. The results indicate that LBP can be used as an adjuvant in the biotherapy of cancer.

Synopsis. Probably the most famous among clinical publications on wolfberries, this often-cited study provides evidence for a positive effect in cancer patients. Significant regression of cancer was noted in patients treated with a tumor-killing agent while taking wolfberries in their diets; this positive effect lasted longer in wolfberry-treated patients.

Although we would like to accept the study as evidence of such simple dietary remedy providing benefit against a major disease, we must be cautious in interpreting these results. Insufficient information is available about the design of the study, such as how long the anti-cancer drugs were given, at what doses, whether more modern anti-cancer agents could have been or were tested, and so on. One major negative effect is the toxicity many patients experience when taking LAK/IL-2. To what degree did the therapy affect appetite and the overall response both to the cancer therapy and the wolfberry intake? We do not even have information on how much wolfberry supplements were provided in the diets of these patients.

This study reveals the problem in interpreting research from Chinese literature—we just do not have enough information, especially from the Methods section of the publication, to intelligently judge such an important study. Therefore, we should treat this and similar results as foundations tempting for further research.

12. **Publication.** Wei Sheng Yan Jiu. 2001 Nov;30(6):333-5. **[Inhibiting the growth of human leukemia cells by Lycium barbarum polysaccharide] [Article in Chinese]** Gan L, Wang J, Zhang S. School of Life Science and Technology, Huazhong University of Science and Technology, Wuhan, China.

Abstract. The effect and the mechanism of Lycium barbarum polysaccharide (LBP) on inhibiting the growth of human leukemia cells were examined. LBP (20, 100, 500, 1000 mg/L) could inhibit the growth of leukemia cells in a dose-dependent manner. Analysis of DNA from the cells treated with LBP revealed a "DNA ladder", showing apoptosis of leukemia cells induced by LBP and perhaps a mechanism of anti-tumorgenesis.

Synopsis. In this study, wolfberry polysaccharides inhibited the growth of human leukemia cells. When DNA of the leukemia cells was analyzed after polysaccharide treatment, there were characteristics of stimulated cell death, or apoptosis. The study provides evidence that wolfberry polysaccharides accelerate the dying of human leukemia cells and so may have immune-stimulating, anti-cancer properties.

13. **Publication.** Zhong Xi Yi Jie He Za Zhi. 1991 Oct;11(10):611-2, 582. **[Radiosensitizing effects of Lycium barbarum polysaccharide for Lewis lung cancer]** [Article in Chinese] Lu CX, Cheng BQ. Cancer Institute, Ningxia Medical College, Yinchuan, China.

Abstract. The radiosensitizing effects of Lycium barbarum polysaccharides (LBP) were observed by the model transplanted Lewis lung cancer on mice. Significant radiosensitizing effects were obtained by combining LBP and radiation.

Synopsis. LBP combines with radiation to sensitize and inhibit the growth of lung cancer cells

14. **Publication.** Planta Med. 2003 Mar;69(3):193-201. **Recent development of antitumor agents from Chinese herbal medicines. Part II. High molecular weight compounds.** Tang W, Hemm I, Bertram B. Department of Chemistry, University of Kaiserslautern, Germany.

Abstract. High molecular weight compounds from Chinese herbal medicines, including ribosome-inactivating proteins and polysaccharides from both fungi and plants, were tested for the treatment of malignant diseases. Polysaccharides possessing immunostimulating activities can be used as adjuvants in tumor treatment. The fungi containing such polysaccharides are usually edible mushrooms or tonics in Traditional Chinese Medicine. Parts from plants such as Radix Astragali and **Fructus Lycii** (wolfberry) containing polysaccharides are mainly used as tonics in Traditional Chinese Medicine.

Synopsis. Wolfberry polysaccharides appear to have anti-neoplastic properties possibly useful in cancer treatment.

Immune-stimulating Properties

15. **Publication.** Zhong Yao Cai. 1999 May;22(5):246-9. **[Effects of pure and crude Lycium barbarum polysaccharides on immunopharmacology]** [Article in Chinese] Luo Q, Yan J, Zhang S. Hubei Medical University, Wuhan, China.

Abstract. Effects of pure Lycium barbarum polysaccharides (LBP) on immunological activity were compared with crude LBP. The pure LBP were divided into different doses, lower doses (5-20 mg/kg.d) of pure LBP showed a remarkable effect on immunological enhancement. Especially, LBP 10 mg/kg.d had a highly significant difference compared with crude LBP on immune indices in mice

Synopsis. This study provided more evidence for unusual immune-stimulating properties of purified wolfberry polysaccharides.

16. **Publication.** Int Immunopharmacol. 2004 Apr;4(4):563-9. **Immunomodulation and anti-tumor activity by a polysaccharide-protein complex from Lycium barbarum.** Gan L, Hua Zhang S, Liang Yang X, Bi Xu H. Institute of Materia Medica, College of Life Science and Technology, Huazhong University of Science and Technology, Wuhan, China.

Abstract. The modulation of a polysaccharide-protein complex from Lycium barbarum (LBP3p) on the immune system in sarcoma-bearing mice was investigated. The mice inoculated with S180 sarcoma cell suspension were treated orally with LBP3p (5, 10 and 20 mg/kg) for 10 days. The effects of LBP3p on transplantable tumors and macrophage phagocytosis, quantitative hemolysis of red blood cells, lymphocyte proliferation, the activity of cytotoxic T lymphocyte, interleukin-2 (IL-2) gene expression and lipid peroxidation were studied. LBP3p could significantly inhibit the growth of transplantable sarcoma S180 cells and increased macrophage phagocytosis. This suggests that LBP3p has a highly significant effect on tumor weight and improves the immune system.

Synopsis. The study provides evidence of several immune - and cell-regulating responses that would provide anti-cancer defenses in mice treated with wolfberry polysaccharide, LBP3p.

17. **Publication.** Eur J Pharmacol. 2003 Jun 27;471(3):217-22. **A polysaccharide-protein complex from Lycium barbarum upregulates cytokine expression in human peripheral blood mononuclear cells.** Gan L, Zhang SH, Liu Q, Xu HB. Institute of Pharmacy, Huazhong University of Science and Technology, Wuhan, China.

Abstract. The production of cytokine is a key event in the initiation and regulation of an immune response. Many compounds are now used routinely to modulate cytokine production, and immune responses in a wide range of diseases, such as cancer. Interleukin-2 and tumor necrosis factor-alpha are two important cytokines in antitumor immunity. In this study, the effects of Lycium barbarum polysaccharide-protein complex (LBP(3p)) on the expression of interleukin-2 and tumor necrosis factor-alpha in human peripheral blood mononuclear cells were investigated by reverse transcription polymerase chain reaction (RT-PCR) and bioassay.

Administration of LBP(3p) increased the expression of interleukin-2 and tumor necrosis factor-alpha at both mRNA and protein levels in a dose-dependent manner. The results suggest that LBP(3p) may induce immune responses and possess potential therapeutic efficacy in cancer.

Synopsis. This study focused on the expression in vitro of interleukin-2 and TNF as indices of the immune response. Wolfberry polysaccharide LBP(3p) increased such expression, indicating that it may enhance immune responsiveness and so may be useful in treating immune-compromised conditions like cancer.

18. **Publication.** Zhong Xi Yi Jie He Xue Bao. 2005 Sep;3(5):374-7.[Effects of Lycium barbarum polysaccharide on tumor microenvironment T-lymphocyte subsets and dendritic cells in H22-bearing mice] [Article in Chinese] He YL, Ying Y, Xu YL, Su JF, Luo H, Wang HF, Department of Pathology, Guangzhou University of Traditional Chinese Medicine, Guangzhou, Guangdong Province, China.

Abstract. The objective of this study was to study the effects of Lycium barbarum polysaccharide (LBP) on tumor microenvironment T-lymphocyte subsets and dendritic cells in H22-bearing mice and the mechanisms for intervention of tumor immune escape by LBP. Methods: H22-bearing mice, a model for cancer, were given LBP orally for two weeks. T-lymphocyte subsets and the phenotypes of dendritic cells in tumor-infiltrating lymphocytes (TIL) were detected by flow cytometry (FCM). Results: LBP could significantly increase the numbers of CD4(+) and CD8(+) T cells in TIL as compared with those in the model control group (P<0.05). In controls, the number of dendritic cells in the tumor microenvironment decreased markedly, while in the LBP-treated group, an increased number of dendritic cells was observed (not statistically significant). Conclusion: LBP may have an anti-tumor effect probably by increasing the numbers of CD4(+) and CD8(+) T cells in TIL. These effects may enhance anti-tumor functions of the immune system.

Synopsis. In this in vitro experiment examining the effects of wolfberry polysaccharides on mouse tumor cells, there was a tendency for positive effects that could have been mediated via immune responses, but the data were not statistically significant.

19. **Publication.** Cancer Biother Radiopharm. 2005 Apr;20(2):155-62.Therapeutic effects of Lycium barbarum polysaccharide (LBP)

on irradiation or chemotherapy-induced myelosuppressive mice. Gong H, Shen P, Jin L, Xing C, Tang F., Capital Medical University, Affiliated Beijing Tiantan Hospital, Beijing, China.

Abstract. The aim of this study was to investigate the effects of Lycium barbarum polysaccharide (LBP) on irradiation—or chemotherapy-induced myelosuppressive mice and cultured peripheral blood mononuclear cells (PBMCs). Methods: In an in vivo experiment, mice were irradiated with a sublethal dose of 550 cGy X-ray or were injected with carboplatin (CB) 125 mg/kg to produce severe myelosuppression. Four to 6 hours after the irradiation or injection, mice were injected with LBP (50, 100, and 200 mg/kg) daily from day 0 to day 6. Blood samples were collected from the tail veins of mice at different time points, and peripheral white blood cells (WBC), red blood cells (RBC), and platelet counts were monitored. Results: Compared to the control, 50 mg/kg LBP (LBP-L) significantly ameliorated the decrease of peripheral WBC of irradiated myelosuppressive mice on day 13, and 100 mg/kg LBP (LBP-M) did the same on days 17 and 21. All dosages of LBP significantly ameliorated the decrease of peripheral RBC of irradiated myelosuppressive mice on days 17 and 25. All dosages of LBP increased peripheral WBC counts of chemotherapy-induced myelosuppressive mice to some extent, but there was no statistical difference when compared to controls. Conclusion: LBP promoted the peripheral blood recovery of irradiation or chemotherapy-induced myelosuppressive mice.

Synopsis. This laboratory study of mice demonstrated that wolfberry polysaccharides had a tendency to decrease white and red blood cell counts occurring with irradiation and chemotherapy (statistically, the results were not significant). Much additional research is needed to prove any usefulness of wolfberries or their extracts in relief from the severe morbidity of cancer or chemotherapies.

Summary of Abstracts on Polysaccharides

Abstracts 1-7 were presented to introduce physicochemical characteristics of wolfberry polysaccharides, allowing insights to their potential for biological actions at the molecular level.

As wolfberry polysaccharides may be similar in structure and function to those in the better-studied Ganoderma mushroom, we presented abstract 8 as a guide to how wolfberry's polysaccharides may influence a variety of health and disease conditions.

Abstracts 9-19 presented some of the research done to date on potential health-promoting properties of wolfberry polysaccharides. Although most of the research is preliminary and inconclusive, the main possible effects of polysaccharides can be summarized as

- antioxidant
- anti-cancer
- stimulating apoptosis
- immune supporting

Despite many years of research interest in wolfberry polysaccharides, the precise cellular and organ effects of this prominent constituent of wolfberries remain vague. To clarify polysaccharide biology, further studies will need to employ conventional bioassay methods, such as structure-activity relationships for each of the putative polysaccharides, receptor identification, binding and inhibitory characteristics, demonstration of specificity and efficacy of physiological actions in controlled systems, and, eventually, pharmacological agonists and antagonists.

In conclusion, although perhaps the "oldest" research area in wolfberry biochemistry, this field remains rudimentary, far from providing clear knowledge of these fascinating and potentially important polysaccharides.

胡萝卜素

CHAPTER 5
Wolfberry Signature Nutrient: Carotenoids

Carotenoid Definitions

We previously introduced the carotenoid class of nutrients in Chapter 3, including concentrations of individual wolfberry carotenoids. As a red-orange berry related in the Solanaceae family to tomatoes, the wolfberry characteristically has high carotenoid content. This class of pigments is an important group of antioxidant nutrients for which an extensive literature is forming about benefits against several diseases.

Before we establish the unusually high content of major carotenoids in wolfberries, we will set the stage with brief definitions and literature showing health benefits of dietary carotenoids.

Carotenoids are sometimes called in science "teraterpenoids" having two classes—carotenes and xanthophylls ("zan-tho-fills"). Carotenes are made up only of hydrogen and carbon atoms whereas xanthophylls also contain oxygen atoms. Beta-carotene and the well-known "tomato antioxidant", lycopene, are typical carotenes. Lutein and zeaxanthin are xanthophylls.

The pink-orange colors of flamingos, goldfish, salmon, pumpkins, bell peppers and autumn leaves are due to carotenoids.

Beta-Carotene

Probably the best known among over 500 carotenoids existing in plants and animals, beta-carotene has the important role of forming base material for synthesis of vitamin A, so is often called a pro-vitamin. Vitamin A is a fat-soluble nutrient found primarily in fish, dairy products, and green, yellow and red vegetables.

Vitamin A is essential for normal growth, regulation of vision, cell structure, bones and teeth, healthy skin, and anti-infective protection of epithelial cells (lining) in the digestive and urinary tracts.

As seen in the previous chapter, beta-carotene belongs to the terpene family that has been shown in studies of Ganoderma mushrooms to have a variety of potential health benefits (Chapter 4).

Zeaxanthin

Zeaxanthin ("zee-a-zan-thin") and lutein are two of the most abundant xanthophyll (oxygen-containing) carotenoids in western diets. Unlike beta-carotene, zeaxanthin is not considered to be a pro-vitamin, as it is not converted in the body into retinol, the active form of vitamin A.

The names of both zeaxanthin and lutein reflect their natural hue— *lutein* is derived from the Latin word *luteus* meaning golden yellow while *zea* refers to the corn genus and *xantho* is derived from a Greek word that means yellow. While these carotenoids both are yellow pigments, they are found concentrated in foods of other colors, notably leafy green vegetables (in which green chlorophyll predominates) and those with red or orange pigments like the wolfberry.

Zeaxanthin is found commonly in egg yolks (about 200 mcg per yolk) and in the petals of deep yellow flowers like marigolds (500 mg per 100 g) that are a major commercial source for zeaxanthin extractions. In Chapter 3, we saw that the total concentration of zeaxanthin in wolfberries—162 mg per 100 g—is perhaps the highest in the world among edible plants.

Beta-cryptoxanthin

Beta-cryptoxanthin ("crip-toe-zan-thin"), classified chemically as a xanthophyll, is one of the most common carotenoids in human diets. It is a provitamin A compound, one of approximately 50 carotenoids converted in the body into retinol. Beta-cryptoxanthin has approximately one-half of the vitamin A activity of beta-carotene.

Lutein

As the stereoisomer of zeaxanthin, lutein ("loo-teen") usually is found in the same plant source with zeaxanthin and serves similar functions in the body. Particularly for retinal and vision support for which lutein and zeaxanthin concentrate as pigments in the retinal macula (below), lutein is perhaps better known among consumers than its close relative zeaxanthin and is a commonly used dietary supplement.

Medical Literature on Carotenoids

Although there is only limited information concerning wolfberry carotenoids having health benefits, reasonable interpretations can be gained from other carotenoid studies in animal disease models and clinical studies in humans. We make these inferences because wolfberries are exceptionally rich sources of 3 main carotenoids—zeaxanthin, beta-carotene and beta-cryptoxanthin. Accordingly, we infer that wolfberries can impart carotenoid benefits as nutrients when included in the diet.

In the following presentation of relevant abstracts from the carotenoid health literature, we indicate the published citation from PubMed (NIH National Library of Medicine) and, if appropriate, provide a synopsis about how results of the study may apply to better understanding of wolfberry's nutritional values.

Health benefits from carotenoids

The following literature was selected to briefly show benefits of dietary carotenoids for the eyes, immune system, cancer, cell functions, antioxidant roles and stroke.

1. **Publication.** Dev Ophthalmol. 2005;38:70-88. **Macular carotenoids: lutein and zeaxanthin.** Stahl W. Heinrich Heine University Dusseldorf, Institute of Biochemistry and Molecular Biology I, Dusseldorf, Germany.

Abstract. The yellow color of the macula lutea is due to the presence of the carotenoid pigments lutein and zeaxanthin. In contrast to human blood and tissues, no other major carotenoids including beta-carotene or lycopene are found in this tissue. The macular carotenoids are suggested to play a role in the protection of the retina against light-induced damage. Epidemiological studies provide some evidence that an *increased consumption of lutein and zeaxanthin from the diet is associated with a lowered risk for age-related macular degeneration,* a disease with increasing incidence in the elderly. Protecting ocular tissue against photooxidative damage carotenoids may act in two ways: first as filters for damaging blue light, and second as antioxidants quenching excited triplet state molecules or singlet molecular oxygen and scavenge further reactive oxygen species like lipid peroxides or the superoxide anion.

Synopsis. This review article discusses the two roles zeaxanthin and lutein have in the retinal macular lutea—1) an antioxidant function for absorbing radical oxygen species and 2) a filtering role to absorb blue light that can damage retinal rods and cones, the "photoreceptors" for vision. As this is an effect of carotenoids worthy of emphasis, we devote a separate section below covering wolfberry benefits for eye health.

2. Publication. J Nutr. 2004 Jan;134(1):257S-261S. **Carotenoid action on the immune response.** Chew BP, Park JS. Department of Animal Sciences, Washington State University, Pullman, WA USA.

Abstract. Early studies demonstrating the ability of dietary carotenes to prevent infections have left open the possibility that the action of these carotenoids may be through their prior conversion to vitamin A. Subsequent studies to demonstrate the specific action of dietary carotenoids have used carotenoids without provitamin A activity such as lutein, canthaxanthin, lycopene and astaxanthin. In fact, these nonprovitamin A carotenoids were as active, and at times more active, than beta-carotene in enhancing cell-mediated and humoral immune response in animals and humans. Another approach to study the possible specific role of dietary carotenoids has used animals that are inefficient converters of carotenoids to vitamin A, for example the domestic cat. Results have similarly shown immuno-enhancement by nonprovitamin A carotenoids, based either on the relative activity or on the type of immune response affected compared to beta-carotene. Certain carotenoids, acting as antioxidants, can potentially reduce the toxic effects of reactive oxygen species (ROS). These ROS, and

WOLFBERRY

therefore carotenoids, have been implicated in the etiology of diseases such as cancer, cardiovascular and neurodegenerative diseases and aging. Recent studies on the role of carotenoids in gene regulation, apoptosis and angiogenesis have advanced our knowledge on the possible mechanism by which carotenoids regulate immune function and cancer.

Synopsis. This review discusses the role of dietary carotenoids as antioxidants reducing the risk or preventing several diseases, including immune disorders, cancer, cardiovascular and neurodegenerative diseases.

3. Publication. J Nutr. 2004 Jan;134(1):225S-230S. From 1989 to 2001: what have we learned about the "biological actions of beta-carotene"? Bendich A. Medical Affairs, GlaxoSmithKline, Parsippany, NJ, USA.

Abstract. Dr. James Allen Olson helped us to define the role of beta-carotene in human health by categorizing these as "functions, actions and associations." In the last decade, significant research has shown that beta-carotene acts as an antioxidant in biologically relevant systems, affects several aspects of human immune function and higher intake/serum levels are associated with improvements in certain physiological functions such as lung function. The unexpected findings of increased lung cancer in beta-carotene supplemented smokers in the ATBC and CARET intervention studies have resulted in the need for expanded research efforts to define the mechanism(s) of action of beta-carotene. Recent survey data as well as laboratory animal studies continue to find an inverse association between beta-carotene and cancer risk. Because beta-carotene is the major source of vitamin A for the majority of the world's population, it is critical to define the safe levels of intake from foods and supplements.

4. Publication. Biol Chem. 2002 Mar-Apr;383(3-4):553-8. Non-antioxidant properties of carotenoids. Stahl W, Ale-Agha N, Polidori MC. Institut fur Physiologische Chemie I, Heinrich-Heine-Universitat Dusseldorf, Germany.

Abstract. Dietary antioxidants such as carotenoids, tocopherols, vitamin C or flavonoids exhibit biological activities that are not directly related to their antioxidant properties. The parent compounds and/or their metabolites have impact on cellular signaling pathways, influence the expression of certain genes or act as inhibitors of regulatory

83

enzymes. Thus, they reveal additional biological effects that might be important for the prevention of degenerative diseases related to the consumption of a diet rich in antioxidants. This review focuses on known non-antioxidant properties of carotenoids, including retinoid-dependent signaling, stimulation of gap junctional communications, impact on the regulation of cell growth and induction of detoxifying enzymes, such as cytochrome P450-dependent monooxygenases.

Synopsis. These authors describe biological roles of carotenoids other than those mentioned most often—the antioxidant and blue light filtering roles. Zeaxanthin, beta-carotene and other carotenoids are involved in 1) cell-to-cell signaling, 2) gene expression, and 3) regulation of several enzymes.

5. Publication. Nutr Clin Care. 2002 Mar-Apr;5(2):56-65. The role of carotenoids in human health. Johnson EJ. Jean Mayer USDA Human Nutrition Research Center on Aging, Tufts University, Boston, MA, USA.

Abstract. Dietary carotenoids are thought to provide health benefits in decreasing the risk of disease, particularly certain cancers and eye disease. The carotenoids that have been most studied in this regard are beta-carotene, lycopene, lutein, and zeaxanthin. In part, the beneficial effects of carotenoids are thought to be due to their role as antioxidants. Beta-carotene may have added benefits due its ability to be converted to vitamin A. Furthermore, lutein and zeaxanthin may be protective in eye disease because they absorb damaging blue light that enters the eye. Food sources of these compounds include a variety of green and yellow fruits and vegetables.

6. Publication. Am J Epidemiol. 2005 Jan 15;161(2):153-160. Plasma carotenoids, retinol, and tocopherols and risk of breast cancer. Tamimi RM, Hankinson SE, Campos H, Spiegelman D, Zhang S, Colditz GA, Willett WC, Hunter DJ. Channing Laboratory, Department of Medicine, Brigham and Women's Hospital and Harvard Medical School, Boston, MA, USA.

Abstract. The roles of carotenoids, retinol, and tocopherols in breast cancer etiology have been inconclusive. The authors prospectively assessed the relations between plasma alpha-carotene, beta-carotene, beta-cryptoxanthin, lycopene, lutein/zeaxanthin, retinol, alpha-tocopherol, and gamma-tocopherol and breast cancer risk by conducting a case-control study using plasma collected from women enrolled in the Nurses' Health Study. A total of 969 cases of breast cancer diagnosed after blood draw and prior to June 1, 1998, were individually matched to controls. The authors conclude that some carotenoids are inversely associated with breast cancer

7. **Publication.** Free Radic Biol Med. 2004 Oct 1;37(7):1018-23. **Is serum gamma-glutamyltransferase inversely associated with serum antioxidants as a marker of oxidative stress?** Lim JS, Yang JH, Chun BY, Kam S, Jacobs DR Jr, Lee DH. Department of Preventive Medicine and Health Promotion Research Center, College of Medicine, Kyungpook National University, Daegu, Korea.

Abstract. A series of studies in black and white women and men have suggested that serum gamma-glutamyltransferase (GGT) within its normal range might be an early marker of oxidative stress. If serum GGT is a marker of oxidative stress, it might have important implications both clinically and epidemiologically. After adjustment for race, sex, age, and total cholesterol, serum concentration of GGT across all deciles was inversely associated with serum concentrations of alpha-carotene, beta-carotene, beta-cryptoxanthin, zeaxanthin/lutein, lycopene, and vitamin C.

8. **Publication.** Stroke. 2004 Jul;35(7):1584-8. **Prospective study of plasma carotenoids and tocopherols in relation to risk of ischemic stroke.** Hak AE, Ma J, Powell CB, Campos H, Gaziano JM, Willett WC, Stampfer MJ. Department of Epidemiology, Harvard School of Public Health, Boston, MA, USA

Abstract. Intake of fruits and vegetables has been related to lower risk of ischemic stroke, but nutrients responsible for this apparent benefit remain ill-defined. Tocopherols (vitamin E) have also been proposed to be protective. Methods: We conducted a prospective, nested case-control analysis among male physicians without diagnosed cardiovascular disease followed-up for up to 13 years in the Physicians' Health Study. Samples from 297 physicians with ischemic stroke were analyzed with paired controls, matched for age and smoking, for 5 major carotenoids (alpha— and beta-carotene, beta-cryptoxanthin, lutein, and lycopene), retinol, and alpha—and gamma-tocopherol. Results: Baseline plasma levels of alpha-carotene and beta-carotene and lycopene tended to be inversely related to risk of ischemic stroke with an apparent threshold effect. Conclusions:

Our data suggest that *higher plasma levels of carotenoids, as markers of fruit and vegetable intake, are inversely related to risk of ischemic stroke* and provide support for recommendations to consume fruits and vegetables regularly.

Summary of this section. The above literature highlights importance of carotenoids for human health. We did not provide complete coverage of available literature that would reveal even broader implications for health values of this nutrient class. Antioxidant functions alone apply to numerous potential health benefits.

The disease areas covered—eye health, immune system, cancer, ischemic stroke—represent significant segments of the population that could benefit from eating carotenoid-rich foods like wolfberries.

Medical Literature on Wolfberry Carotenoids

Below, we present 7 studies specifically on wolfberry carotenoids, including analyses of carotenoid isolation, bioavailability after wolfberry consumption, and potential liver protection.

9. **Publication.** Se Pu. 1998 Jul;16(4):341-3. **[Separation and determination of carotenoids in Fructus lycii by isocratic non-aqueous reversed-phase liquid chromatography]** [Article in Chinese] Li Z, Peng G, Zhang S. Department of Food Science & Technology, Huazhong Agricultural University, Wuhan, China.

Abstract. High performance liquid chromatography using a non-aqueous reversed phase with isocratic elution of C18 columns is a powerful tool for investigating the carotenoid composition of Fructus Lycii. This paper compared the effect of different eluents on the separation of carotenoids. Ten carotenoids were separated from Fructus Lycii. Fructus Lycii contains 2952 micrograms/g of total carotenoids, but 98.6% of carotenoids are existed as esterified forms, zeaxanthin dipalmitate are accounted for 77.5% of the total.

Synopsis. 10 carotenoids from wolfberries were isolated although not presented individually with data in this abstract. The results showed that they were mainly in the form of esters totaling 2952 mcg per gram and that zeaxanthin dipalmitate comprised 77.5% or 2290 mcg per gram of the total carotenoid content in wolfberries.

10. **Publication.** Br J Nutr. 2005 Jan;93(1):123-30. **Fasting plasma zeaxanthin response to Fructus barbarum L. (wolfberry; Kei Tze) in a food-based human supplementation trial.** Cheng CY,

Chung WY, Szeto YT, Benzie IF. Antioxidant Research Group, Faculty of Health and Social Sciences, The Hong Kong Polytechnic University, Kowloon, Hong Kong SAR, China.

Abstract. Age-related macular degeneration (AMD) is a common disorder that causes irreversible loss of central vision. Increased intake of foods containing zeaxanthin may be effective in preventing AMD because the macula accumulates zeaxanthin and lutein, oxygenated carotenoids with antioxidant and blue light-absorbing properties. Lycium barbarum L. is a small red berry known as Fructus lycii and wolfberry in the West, and Kei Tze and Gou Qi Zi in Asia. Wolfberry is rich in zeaxanthin dipalmitate, and is valued in Chinese culture for being good for vision. The aim of this study, which was a single-blinded, placebo-controlled, human intervention trial of parallel design, was to provide data on how fasting plasma zeaxanthin concentration changes as a result of dietary supplementation with whole wolfberries. Fasting blood was collected from healthy, consenting subjects; fourteen subjects took 15 g/d wolfberry (estimated to contain almost 3 mg zeaxanthin) for 28 d. Repeat fasting blood was collected on day 29. Age—and sex-matched controls (n 13) took no wolfberry. Responses in the two groups were compared using the Mann-Whitney test. After supplementation, plasma zeaxanthin increased 2.5-fold: mean values on day 1 and 29 were 0.038 (sem 0.003) and 0.096 (sem 0.009) micromol/l (P<0.01), respectively, for the supplementation group; and 0.038 (sem 0.003) and 0.043 (sem 0.003) micromol/l (P>0.05), respectively, for the control group. This human supplementation trial shows that zeaxanthin in whole wolfberries is bioavailable and that intake of a modest daily amount markedly increases fasting plasma zeaxanthin levels. These new data will support further study of dietary strategies to maintain macular pigment density.

Synopsis. This straightforward but important study focused on the ability of wolfberry intake to be translated into detectable blood levels of zeaxanthin. Subjects ate 15 grams of wolfberries per day for 28 days after which zeaxanthin blood levels more than doubled compared to controls who did not eat wolfberries. The experiment shows that eating wolfberries makes zeaxanthin levels increase substantially in the blood and indicates that blood levels of this important carotenoid can be easily increased by including wolfberries in the diet.

11. Publication. Br J Nutr. 2004 May;91(5):707-13. Comparison of

plasma responses in human subjects after the ingestion of 3R,3R'-zeaxanthin dipalmitate from wolfberry (Lycium barbarum) and non-esterified 3R,3R'-zeaxanthin using chiral high-performance liquid chromatography. Breithaupt DE, Weller P, Wolters M, Hahn A. Institute for Food Chemistry, University of Hohenheim, Stuttgart, Germany.

Abstract. Age-related macular degeneration (AMD) is one of the most common eye diseases of elderly individuals. It has been suggested that lutein and zeaxanthin may reduce the risk for AMD. Information concerning the absorption of non-esterified or esterified zeaxanthin is rather scarce. Furthermore, the formation pathway of meso (3R,3'S)-zeaxanthin, which does not occur in plants but is found in the macula, has not yet been identified. Thus, the present study was designed to assess the concentration of 3R,3R'-zeaxanthin reached in plasma after the consumption of a single dose of native 3R,3'R-zeaxanthin palmitate from wolfberry (Lycium barbarum) or non-esterified 3R,3'R-zeaxanthin in equal amounts. In a randomised, single-blind cross-over study, twelve volunteers were administered non-esterified or esterified 3R,3'R-zeaxanthin (5 mg) suspended in yoghurt together with a balanced breakfast. After fasting overnight, blood was collected before the dose (0 h), and at 3, 6, 9, 12, and 24 h after the dose. The concentration of non-esterified 3R,3'R-zeaxanthin was determined by high-performance liquid chromatography. Independent of the consumed diet, plasma 3R,3'R-zeaxanthin concentrations increased significantly and peaked after 9-24 h. Thus, the study indicates an enhanced bioavailability of 3R,3'R-zeaxanthin dipalmitate compared with the non-esterified form.

Synopsis. Zeaxanthin levels, in the ester form preferred for uptake by the retina, increased in blood after a single meal dose of wolfberries. The results indicate prompt availability of wolfberry zeaxanthin after consumption for uptake in the retina of the eye or other organs.

12. Publication. J Agric Food Chem. 2003 Nov 19;51(24):7044-9. Identification and quantification of zeaxanthin esters in plants using liquid chromatography-mass spectrometry. Weller P, Breithaupt DE. Universitat Hohenheim, Institut fur Lebensmittelchemie, Stuttgart, Germany.

Abstract. It has been suggested that lutein and zeaxanthin may decrease the risk for age-related macular degeneration. Surprisingly, oleoresins rich in zeaxanthin are not yet available on the market. Several authors have reported enhanced stability of esterified xanthophylls, so plants containing zeaxanthin esters were investigated to establish valuable sources for the production of durable oleoresins. Liquid chromatography-atmospheric pressure chemical ionization mass spectrometry [LC-(APCI)MS] was used to unequivocally identify zeaxanthin esters of a standard mixture and in several plant extracts. Dried wolfberries (Lycium barbarum), Chinese lanterns (Physalis alkekengi), orange pepper (Capsicum annuum), and sea buckthorn (Hippophae rhamnoides) proved to be valuable zeaxanthin ester sources.

Synopsis. Useful sources of zeaxanthin esters for potential production of oleoresins that could be further developed into extracts for food or medical applications include wolfberry and another berry native to China, seabuckthorn.

13. Publication. Invest Ophthalmol Vis Sci. 2001 Feb;42(2):466-71. **Absorption and tissue distribution of zeaxanthin and lutein in rhesus monkeys after taking Fructus lycii (Gou qi zi) extract.** Leung I, Tso M, Li W, Lam T. Department of Ophthalmology and Visual Sciences, The Chinese University of Hong Kong.

Abstract. Purpose: To study serum and tissue levels of zeaxanthin and lutein after feeding rhesus monkeys an extract of Fructus lycii (gou qi zi). Methods: A carotenoid-containing fraction (P1) from an extract of F. lycii (equivalent to 2.2 mg zeaxanthin) was fed to three rhesus monkeys for 6 weeks as a daily dietary supplement through a nasogastric tube. Three other monkeys were fed with the vehicle (olive oil) similarly for 4 weeks as a control. Another three animals were fed with normal diet only. Tissue samples were analyzed for zeaxanthin and lutein by high-pressure liquid chromatography. Results: Serum levels of zeaxanthin and lutein in the P1-fed group were significantly higher than those of vehicle control ($P<0.05$). Besides the retina, the liver had the highest zeaxanthin and lutein levels, whereas the levels in the brain were undetectable. P1 supplement appeared to elevate zeaxanthin levels in liver and spleen. P1 treatment elevated zeaxanthin density but not lutein in the macula. Conclusions: Macular density of zeaxanthin was raised by feeding a carotenoid-containing fraction of F. lycii. Therefore, F. lycii is a good dietary source of zeaxanthin supplement.

Synopsis. Oral dosing of monkeys with a carotenoid extract from wolfberries increased zeaxanthin and lutein levels in the retinas, spleens and livers but not in the brains of monkeys. The study indicates that consuming wolfberries would be an effective way to elevate zeaxanthin levels in the body, especially in the retinal macula lutea.

14. **Publication.** Biol Pharm Bull. 2002 Mar;25(3):390-2. **Zeaxanthin dipalmitate from Lycium chinense fruit reduces experimentally induced hepatic fibrosis in rats.** Kim HP, Lee EJ, Kim YC, Kim J, Kim HK, Park JH, Kim SY, Kim YC. College of Pharmacy, Seoul National University, Korea.

Abstract. We previously reported that zeaxanthin dipalmitate (ZD), a carotenoid from Lycium chinense fruit, reduces myofibroblast-like cell proliferation and collagen synthesis in vitro. To determine whether ZD might reduce the severity of hepatic fibrosis in an animal model, hepatic fibrosis was induced in rats by bile duct ligation/scission (BDL) for a period of 6 weeks. Treatment of BDL rats with ZD at a dose of 25 mg/kg body weight significantly reduced the activities of aspartate transaminase (p<0.05) and alkaline phosphatase (p<0.001) in serum. Furthermore, collagen deposition was significantly reduced. These results showed that ZD effectively inhibited hepatic fibrosis in BDL rats, at least in part via its antioxidative activity.

Synopsis. In a rat model of liver fibrosis disease, zeaxanthin from wolfberries reduced the activities of two liver enzymes (provided protection) and the amount of liver collagen formed (inhibited the fibrosis). The authors speculated that zeaxanthin's antioxidant properties provided these beneficial effects.

15. **Publication.** Res Commun Mol Pathol Pharmacol. 1997 Sep;97(3):301-14. **Zeaxanthin dipalmitate from Lycium chinense has hepatoprotective activity.** Kim HP, Kim SY, Lee EJ, Kim YC, Kim YC. College of Pharmacy, Seoul National University, Korea.

Abstract. We previously reported the isolation of zeaxanthin and zeaxanthin dipalmitate using bioactivity-guided fractionation to discover hepatoprotective components of Lycium chinense against carbon tetrachloride induced hepatotoxicity. The present study was designed to uncover the effects of zeaxanthin dipalmitate on liver cells in vitro. The effects of zeaxanthin dipalmitate on the formation of nitric oxide (NO) and the release of tumor necrosis factor-alpha (TNF-alpha) from Kupffer cells and peritoneal macrophages were assayed. Zeaxanthin dipalmitate showed significant liver protection against carbon tetrachloride toxicity. Zeaxanthin dipalmitate reduced collagen synthesis by 65.1% (p < 0.05) as compared to untreated controls. The formation of NO in either Kupffer cells or in peritoneal macrophages was significantly decreased by zeaxanthin dipalmitate in a concentration dependent manner. From these results, we conclude that zeaxanthin dipalmitate exerts potent liver protection by inhibiting cell proliferation and collagen synthesis.

Synopsis. Zeaxanthin from wolfberries protected rat liver cells in vitro from oxidative damage produced by toxicity and from developing fibrosis. Zeaxanthin inhibited formation of nitric oxide, a free radical, and prevented the proliferation of cells resulting from toxic stimulation by carbon tetrachloride.

Summary: Wolfberry Carotenoids

Wolfberry carotenoids have been studied to reveal properties of their behavior in the body after consuming the fruit. 77% of wolfberry carotenoids exist as zeaxanthin, a carotenoid source shown to be effective as an antioxidant. Protection of liver cells exposed to toxins is an established finding of Chinese wolfberry research, as well as zeaxanthin being a preferred substrate for uptake by the macula lutea of the eye where it shields retinal photoreceptors from the damaging effects of intense sunlight.

Common among the probable health benefits of carotenoid intake through the diet is broad physiological protection afforded by antioxidant nutrients. Accordingly, we provide a view now of this important phytochemical class to which many of wolfberry's constituents belong.

Carotenoids as Antioxidant Nutrients in Health and Disease

It is appropriate that we discuss this subject here as wolfberries are perhaps best known already in public information as high-antioxidant food. Above and in Chapters 2 and 3, we learned that wolfberries contain a variety of phytochemicals that may apply to antioxidant quality, namely

- Carotenoids, pigmented phytochemicals characterizing wolfberry's red-orange color. Including beta-carotene, beta-cryptoxanthin and zeaxanthin/lutein, carotenoids quench free radicals, i.e., provide electrons that render radical chemical species neutral or absorb radicals into their chemical structure to inactivate the radical

- Vitamins, A, C and E, have several antioxidant functions in the body
- "Antioxidant" minerals—zinc, copper, manganese, magnesium and selenium—have numerous roles as cofactors for antioxidant enzymes.

Below, we shall first review discussions in the medical literature that have linked these antioxidant nutrients to health. Doing so, we explore their potential roles in prevention or treatment of several diseases, including cancer, heart and vascular disorders, macular degeneration of aging, chronic inflammation and pulmonary disorders.

16. Publication. Public Health Nutr. 2004 May;7(3):407-22. **A review of the epidemiological evidence for the 'antioxidant hypothesis'.** Stanner SA, Hughes J, Kelly CN, Buttriss J. British Nutrition Foundation, London, UK.

Abstract. The British Nutrition Foundation was recently commissioned by the Food Standards Agency to conduct a review of the government's research programme on Antioxidants in Food. Part of this work involved an independent review of the scientific literature on the role of antioxidants in chronic disease prevention, which is presented in this paper. There is consistent evidence that diets rich in fruit and vegetables and other plant foods are associated with moderately lower overall mortality rates and lower death rates from cardiovascular disease and some types of cancer. *The 'antioxidant hypothesis' proposes that vitamin C, vitamin E, carotenoids and other antioxidant nutrients afford protection against chronic diseases by decreasing oxidative damage.* Although scientific rationale and observational studies have been convincing, randomized primary and secondary intervention trials have failed to show any consistent benefit from the use of antioxidant supplements on cardiovascular disease or cancer risk, with some trials even suggesting possible harm in certain subgroups. These trials have usually involved the administration of single antioxidant nutrients given at relatively high doses. The results of trials investigating the effect of a balanced combination of antioxidants at levels achievable by diet are awaited. Conclusion: The suggestion that antioxidant supplements can prevent chronic diseases has not been proved or consistently supported by the findings of published intervention trials. Further evidence regarding the efficacy, safety and appropriate dosage of antioxidants in relation to chronic disease is needed. The most prudent public health advice remains to increase the consumption of plant foods, as such dietary patterns are associated with reduced risk of chronic disease.

17. Publication. Biomed Pharmacother. 2004 Mar;58(2):100-10. **The role of carotenoids in the prevention of human pathologies.** Tapiero H, Townsend DM, Tew KD. Universite de Paris-Faculte de Pharmacie CNRS UMR, Chatenay Malabry, France.

Abstract. Reactive oxygen species (ROS) and oxidative damage to biomolecules have been postulated to be involved in the causation and progression of several chronic diseases, including cancer and cardiovascular diseases, the two major causes of morbidity and mortality in the Western world. Consequently dietary antioxidants, which inactivate ROS and provide protection from oxidative damage are being considered as important preventive strategic molecules. Carotenoids have been implicated as important dietary nutrients having antioxidant potential, being involved in the scavenging of two of the ROS, singlet molecular oxygen and peroxyl radicals generated in the process of lipid peroxidation. Carotenoids are lipophilic molecules which tend to accumulate in lipophilic compartments like membranes or lipoproteins. Chronic ethanol consumption significantly increases hydrogen peroxide and decreases mitochondrial glutathione (GSH) in cells. The depletion of mitochondrial GSH and the rise of hydrogen peroxide are responsible for ethanol-induced apoptosis. Increased intake of lycopene, a major carotenoid in tomatoes, consumed as the all-trans-isomer attenuates alcohol induced apoptosis and reduces risk of prostate, lung and digestive cancers. *Cancer-preventive activities of carotenoids have been associated as well as with their antioxidant properties and the induction and stimulation of intercellular communication* via gap junctions which play a role in the regulation of cell growth, differentiation and apoptosis.

18. Publication. Curr Eye Res. 2004 Dec;29(6):387-401. **AMD and micronutrient antioxidants.** Hogg R, Chakravarthy U. Ophthalmology & Vision Science, Institute of Clinical Science, The Royal Victoria Hospital, Belfast, Northern Ireland.

Abstract. Age-related maculopathy (ARM) is a common clinical entity. The late-stage manifestations of ARM, which are known as age-related macular degeneration (AMD), have devastating consequences for vision. Various risk factors have been identified in the development of the condition, which are consistent with the premise that oxidative stress plays an important role in its pathogenesis. Thus, the possibility that antioxidant balance can be manipulated through diet or supplementation has created much interest. Associations between diet and nutrition and the clinical features of ARM have been described. Scrutiny of the literature shows consistency in the report of notable reductions in serum micronutrients in wet AMD, however, the evidence for causation is still circumstantial. In this comprehensive review of the clinical literature, we have assessed the evidence for a link between diet and nutrition as risk factors for the development of ARM and AMD. All published case control, population-based, and interventional studies on ARM were examined. Although initial support appeared to be moderate and somewhat contradictory, the evidence that lifetime oxidative stress plays an important role in the development of ARM is now compelling. The positive outcomes in the Age-Related Eye Diseases Study, a major controlled clinical trial, have given hope that *modulation of the antioxidant balance through supplementation can help prevent progression of ARM to AMD.*

19. **Publication.** J Nutr. 2003 Mar;133 Suppl 3:933S-940S. **Antioxidant nutrients and chronic disease: use of biomarkers of exposure and oxidative stress status in epidemiologic research.** Mayne ST. Department of Epidemiology and Public Health, Yale University School of Medicine and Yale Cancer Center, New Haven, CT, USA

Abstract. Oxidation of lipid, nucleic acids or protein has been suggested to be involved in the etiology of several chronic diseases including cancer, cardiovascular disease, cataract, age-related macular degeneration and aging in general. A large body of research has investigated the potential role of antioxidant nutrients in the prevention of these and other chronic diseases. This review concentrates on the following *antioxidant nutrients: beta-carotene and other carotenoids, vitamin E, vitamin C and selenium.* The first part of the review emphasizes the utility of biological markers of exposure for these nutrients and the relationship to dietary intake data. The second part considers functional assays of oxidative stress status in humans including the strengths and limitations of various assays available for use in epidemiologic research. The review concludes with a discussion of methodological issues and challenges for studies involving biomarkers of exposure to antioxidant nutrients and of oxidative stress status.

20. **Publication.** J Am Pharm Assoc (Wash). 2000 Nov-Dec;40(6):785-99. **Antioxidant nutrients: current dietary recommendations and research update.** McDermott JH, School of Pharmacy, University of North Carolina, Chapel Hill, USA.

Abstract. To review the importance of antioxidant nutrients in the maintenance of health and the prevention and treatment of disease, with a focus on data pertaining to vitamin C, vitamin E, selenium, and carotenoids. A secondary objective was to discuss the new Dietary Reference Intakes released by the Institute of Medicine (IOM) for these nutrients. IOM reports on the use of antioxidant vitamins were reviewed for nutrient recommendations. In addition, a Medline search was performed to identify recent research and review articles on the topic, which were analyzed to identify key research findings in the area. The review discusses the biologic processes of oxidation reactions and antioxidants in biologic systems, provides an overview of information on selected antioxidant nutrients, and explores their role in the prevention and treatment of cancer, cardiovascular disease, ocular disorders, and respiratory disorders. Conclusion: There appear to be *significant health benefits from dietary antioxidants,* as can be found in fruits and vegetables.

21. **Publication.** Clin Nutr. 2005 Apr;24(2):172-83. **Can oxidative damage be treated nutritionally?** Berger MM. Surgical ICU, Soins Intensifs Chirurgicaux et Centre des Brules, Lausanne, Switzerland.

Abstract. Background & aims: Nutrition and dietary patterns have been shown to have direct impact on health of the population and of selected patient groups. The beneficial effects have been attributed to the reduction of oxidative damage caused by the normal or excessive free radical production. The papers aims at collecting evidence of successful supplementation strategies Methods: Review of the literature reporting on antioxidant supplementation trials in the general population and critically ill patients. Results: *Antioxidant vitamin and trace element intakes have been shown to be particularly important in the prevention of cancer, cardiovascular diseases, age related ocular diseases and in aging.* In animal models, targeted interventions have been associated with reduction of tissue destruction is brain and myocardium ischemia-reperfusion models. In the critically ill antioxidant supplements have resulted in reduction of organ failure and of infectious complications.

Conclusions: Antioxidant micronutrients have beneficial effects in defined models and pathologies of the general population and in critical illnesses. Ongoing research encourages this supportive therapeutic approach. Further research is required to determine the optimal micronutrient combinations and the doses required according to timing of intervention.

Carotenoids and Eye Health

Perhaps the most compelling justification for dietary carotenoids comes from the literature on eye health, particularly with regard to macular pigmentation provided specifically by zeaxanthin and lutein. It is clear from reports over the last few years that these two carotenoids are absorbed selectively into the retinal macula where they furnish dual protection—an antioxidant role combined with a filtering function to dampen the intensity of blue light. Without sufficient carotenoids in the diet, these pigmentation levels presumably are low, permitting the damaging effects of age-related macular degeneration.

The retinal macula lutea is a model system for how specifically wolfberry nutrients may benefit human eye health. The retinal macula lutea is the eye region in which light is transformed via photoreceptors into neuroelectrical signals for interpreting vision.

In the retinal fovea and macula, the carotenoids zeaxanthin and lutein are preferentially stored and integrated into yellow macular pigment that serves the two functions mentioned above: to filter and absorb intense light and to provide a carotenoid-enriched antioxidant reserve for neutralizing radical oxygen species.

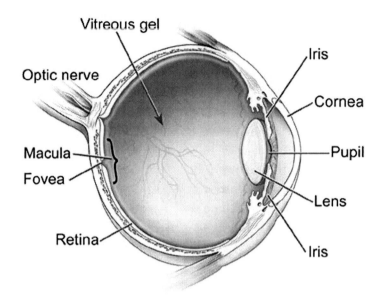

Courtesy of National Eye Institute, National Institutes of Health, Bethesda, MD

Our purpose now is to lay a foundation for this important beneficial effect of wolfberry carotenoids by reviewing literature on the nutrients of ocular health.

22. Publication. Ophthalmic Physiol Opt. 2004 Jul;24(4):339-49. **An ideal ocular nutritional supplement?** Bartlett H, Eperjesi F. Neurosciences Research Institute, School of Life and Health Sciences, Aston University, Birmingham, UK.

Abstract. The role of nutritional supplementation in prevention of onset or progression of ocular disease is of interest to health care professionals and patients. The aim of this review is to identify those antioxidants most appropriate for inclusion in an ideal ocular nutritional supplement, suitable for those with a family history of glaucoma, cataract, or age-related macular disease, or lifestyle factors predisposing onset of these conditions, such as smoking, poor nutritional status, or high levels of sunlight exposure. It would also be suitable for those with early stages of age-related ocular disease. Literature searches were carried out on Web of Science and PubMed for articles relating to the use of nutrients in ocular disease. Those highlighted for possible inclusion were *vitamins A, B, C and E, carotenoids beta-carotene, lutein, and zeaxanthin, minerals selenium and zinc, and the herb, Ginkgo biloba.* Conflicting evidence is presented for vitamins A and E in prevention of ocular disease; these vitamins have roles in the production of rhodopsin and prevention of lipid peroxidation respectively. B vitamins have been linked with a reduced risk of cataract and studies have provided evidence supporting a protective role of vitamin C in cataract prevention. Beta-carotene is active in the prevention of free radical formation, but has been linked with an increased risk of lung cancer in smokers. Improvements in visual function in patients with age-related macular disease have been noted with lutein and zeaxanthin supplementation. Selenium has been linked with a reduced risk of cataract and activates the antioxidant enzyme glutathione peroxidase, protecting cell membranes from oxidative damage while zinc, although an essential component of antioxidant enzymes, has been highlighted for risk of adverse effects. As well as reducing platelet aggregation and increasing vasodilation, Gingko biloba has been linked with improvements in pre-existing field damage in some patients with normal tension glaucoma. *We advocate that vitamins C and E, and lutein/zeaxanthin should be included in our theoretically ideal ocular nutritional supplement.*

23. **Publication.** Surv Ophthalmol. 2005 Mar-Apr;50(2):183-93. **The macular xanthophylls.** Ahmed SS, Lott MN, Marcus DM. Department of Ophthalmology, Medical College of Georgia, Augusta, GA, USA.

Abstract. The macular pigments are predominantly composed of three carotenoids: lutein, zeaxanthin, and meso-zeaxanthin. These carotenoids are concentrated and distributed in a selective manner. The properties of these pigments are further explored along with their methods of uptake, stabilization, and storage. The dual nature of these pigments as filters and antioxidants are elaborated upon in relation to their protective effects upon the macula, specifically in age-related macular degeneration. Evidence suggests that increased levels of macular pigment are correlated with a decreased risk of age-related macular degeneration. Many have sought to exploit this therapeutic relation. Studies reveal that *oral supplementation with lutein and zeaxanthin can increase the levels of macular pigments in the retina and plasma.* The effects of such supplementation on actual ocular function have yet to be fully addressed. New and standardized methods of assessing macular pigment density are discussed and future areas of research to further our understanding of macular xanthophylls as they pertain to age-related macular degeneration are highlighted.

24. **Publication.** Prog Retin Eye Res. 2002 Mar;21(2):225-40. **Macular pigment: influences on visual acuity and visibility.** Wooten BR, Hammond BR. Walter S. Hunter Laboratory, Brown University, Providence, RI

Abstract. There is increasing evidence that the macular pigment (MP) carotenoids lutein (L) and zeaxanthin (Z) protect the retina and lens from age-related loss. As a result, the use of L and Z supplements has increased dramatically in recent years. An increasing number of reports have suggested that L and Z supplementation (and increased MP density) are related to improved visual performance in normal subjects and patients with retinal and lenticular disease. These improvements in vision could be due either to changes in the underlying biology and/or optical changes. The optical mechanisms, i.e., preferential absorption of short-wave light, underlying these putative improvements in vision, however, have not been properly evaluated.

Two major hypotheses are discussed. The acuity hypothesis posits that MP could improve visual function by reducing the effects of chromatic aberration. The visibility hypothesis is based on the idea that *MP may improve vision through the atmosphere by preferentially absorbing blue haze* (short-wave dominant light that produces a veiling luminance when viewing objects at a distance).

Age-Related Eye Disease Study, AREDS

In Chapter 2, we introduced the term "clinical trial" and emphasized that such a rigorous study in humans is essential for regulatory approval of drugs and nutrients having specific health claims. For nutrient-related eye health and wolfberry carotenoids, the following presentation of the AREDS report is significant since this 10-year study of more than 3000 people showed benefit of nutrients (found in wolfberries) against the progression of age-related macular degeneration.

25. **Publication.** Arch Ophthalmol. 2001 Oct;119(10):1417-36. **A randomized, placebo-controlled, clinical trial of high-dose supplementation with vitamins C and E, beta carotene, and zinc**

for age-related macular degeneration and vision loss. Age-Related Eye Disease Study Research Group, US National Eye Institute, National Institutes of Health.

Comment. In this landmark study of nutrients important for protecting eye health in age-related disorders such as macular degeneration, *high daily doses of vitamins C and E, beta-carotene and the mineral zinc were shown to significantly reduce rates of vision loss in people age 55 years and older.* Discussion in the AREDS report mentioned the potential value of carotenoids, zeaxanthin and lutein, which were not included at the time of study only because of unavailable formulations and/or lack of guidance on doses. Diseases of the eye lens, e.g., cataract, appear not to be affected by antioxidant nutrients, as these disorders tend to be inevitable with aging.

Considerable follow up on this research over the past 4 years emphasizes the probable value to vision of a diet high in antioxidant nutrients, emphasizing this combination of vitamins, carotenoids and zinc—all of which are present in high concentrations in wolfberries (although not in amounts equal to those of the AREDS study).

Below, we review additional literature highlighting carotenoids especially recognized as favorable for reducing the risk of vision loss during aging.

26. Publication. Toxicol Lett. 2004 Apr 15;150(1):57-83. The science behind lutein. Alves-Rodrigues A, Shao A. Research and Development Department, Kemin Foods Europe, Lisbon, Portugal.

Abstract. In humans, as in plants, the xanthophyll lutein is believed to function in two important ways: first as a filter of high energy blue light, and second as an antioxidant that quenches and scavenges photo induced reactive oxygen species (ROS). Evidence suggests that lutein consumption is inversely related to eye diseases such as age-related macular degeneration (AMD) and cataracts. This is supported by the finding that lutein (and its stereo isomer, zeaxanthin) are deposited in the lens and the macula lutea, an area of the retina responsible for central and high acuity vision. Human intervention studies show that lutein supplementation results in increased macular pigment and improved vision in patients with AMD and other ocular diseases. Lutein may also serve to protect skin from UV-induced damage and may help reduce the risk of cardiovascular disease.

Crystalline lutein is readily absorbed from foods and from dietary supplements whereas, to enter the bloodstream, lutein esters require prior de-esterification by intestinal enzymes. Unlike the hydrocarbon carotenoids which are mainly found in the LDL fraction, xanthophylls like lutein and zeaxanthin are incorporated into both HDL and LDL. Today, lutein can be obtained from the diet in several different ways, including via supplements, and most recently in functional foods. Animal toxicology studies have been performed to established lutein's safety as a nutrient. These studies have contributed to the classification of purified crystalline lutein as generally recognized as safe (GRAS). The achievement of GRAS status for purified crystalline lutein allows for the addition of this form into several food and beverage applications.

27. **Publication.** Asia Pac J Clin Nutr. 2003;12 Suppl:S5. **Nutritional factors in the development of age-related eye disease.** Mitchell P, Smith W, Cumming RG, Flood V, Rochtchina E, Wang JJ. University of Sydney Department of Ophthalmology, Westmead Hospital, Sydney (Westmead Millennium Institute, Centre for Vision Research), Australia.

Abstract. Nutritional associations have been found with two major eye diseases, age-related macular degeneration (AMD), the leading causes of severe visual impairment (blindness) and cataract, a cause of mild to moderate visual impairment. These data have derived from population-based studies of older communities and samples, clinic-based case-control studies, and from the findings of a recent, large randomized clinical trial; the Age Related Eye Disease Study (AREDS). For AMD, some population-based and case-control studies suggested protective roles for diet or supplementary zinc and antioxidants, although these data have been variable and relatively inconsistent. Benefit, however, was confirmed in the AREDS trial, which demonstrated, over 6 years, up to a 25% reduction in development of advanced disease or severe visual impairment in the group taking large, combined doses of zinc and vitamins A (as beta-carotene), C and E. There is now also increasing circumstantial evidence for *beneficial effects from the xanthophyll carotenoids, lutein and zeaxanthin*, which were not incorporated in the AREDS supplement. Many studies have also shown protective effects on AMD from reduced dietary saturated fat and regular consumption of fish. For cataract, although earlier studies suggested potential benefits from increased dietary intakes of antioxidants, no benefit from supplements was confirmed in the AREDS trial.

28. Publication. Nutr J. 2003 Dec 11;2(1):20. **The role of the carotenoids, lutein and zeaxanthin, in protecting against age-related macular degeneration: A review based on controversial evidence.** Mozaffarieh M, Sacu S, Wedrich A. Department of Ophthalmology, University of Vienna, Austria.

Abstract. Purpose: A review of the role of the carotenoids, lutein and zeaxanthin, and their function in altering the pathogenesis of age-related macular degeneration (AMD). Medline and Embase searches were used. Recent evidence introduces the possibility that lutein and zeaxanthin, carotenoids found in a variety of fruits and vegetables may protect against the common eye disease of macular degeneration. This potential and the lack to slow the progression of macular degeneration, has fueled high public interest in the health benefits of these carotenoids and prompted their inclusion in various supplements. The body of evidence supporting a role in this disease ranges from basic studies in experimental animals to various other clinical and epidemiological studies. Conclusion: *An intake of dietary supplied nutrients rich in the carotenoids, lutein and zeaxanthin, appears to be beneficial in protecting retinal tissues,* but this is not proven. Until scientifically sound knowledge is available we recommend for patients judged to be at risk for AMD to: alter their diet to more dark green leafy vegetables, wear UV protective lenses and a hat when outdoors.

29. Publication. J Am Coll Nutr. 2000 Oct;19(5 Suppl):522S-527S. **The potential role of dietary xanthophylls in cataract and age-related macular degeneration.** Moeller SM, Jacques PF, Blumberg JB. Jean Mayer USDA Human Nutrition Research Center on Aging, Tufts University, Boston, MA

Abstract. The carotenoid xanthophylls, lutein and zeaxanthin, accumulate in the eye lens and macular region of the retina. Lutein and zeaxanthin concentrations in the macula are greater than those found in plasma and other tissues. A relationship between macular pigment optical density, a marker of lutein and zeaxanthin concentration in the macula, and lens optical density, an antecedent of cataractous changes, has been suggested. The xanthophylls may act to protect the eye from ultraviolet phototoxicity via quenching reactive oxygen species and/or other mechanisms. Some observational studies have shown that generous intakes of lutein and zeaxanthin, particularly from certain xanthophyll-rich foods like spinach, broccoli and eggs, are associated with a significant reduction in the risk for cataract (up to 20%) and for age-related macular degeneration (up to 40%). While the pathophysiology of cataract and age-related macular degeneration is complex and contains both environmental and genetic components, research studies suggest *dietary factors including antioxidant vitamins and xanthophylls may contribute to a reduction in the risk of these degenerative eye diseases.*

The health effects of dietary carotenoids should not be limited to eye benefits, as there is a considerable literature reviewed at both the opening and close of this chapter for several other diseases. Specific example—these following studies that show beneficial effects of carotenoids on cancer.

30. **Publication.** Integr Cancer Ther. 2004 Dec;3(4):333-41. **Dietary antioxidants and human cancer.** Borek C. Department of Community Health and Family Medicine, Nutrition Infectious Disease Unit, Tufts University School of Medicine, Boston, MA.

Abstract. Epidemiological studies show that a high intake of anti-oxidant-rich foods is inversely related to cancer risk. While animal and cell cultures confirm the anticancer effects of antioxidants, intervention trials to determine their ability to reduce cancer risk have been inconclusive, although selenium and vitamin E reduced the risk of some forms of cancer, including prostate and colon cancer, and carotenoids have been shown to help reduce breast cancer risk. Cancer treatment by radiation and anticancer drugs reduces inherent antioxidants and induces oxidative stress, which increases with disease progression. Vitamins E and C have been shown to ameliorate adverse side effects associated with free radical damage to normal cells in cancer therapy, such as mucositis and fibrosis, and to reduce the recurrence of breast cancer. While clinical studies on the effect of anti-oxidants in modulating cancer treatment are limited in number and size, experimental studies show that *antioxidant vitamins and some phytochemicals selectively induce apoptosis in cancer cells but not in normal cells and prevent angiogenesis and metastatic spread, suggesting a potential role for antioxidants as adjuvants in cancer therapy.*

31. **Publication.** J Agric Food Chem. 2004 Dec 1;52(24):7264-71. **Inhibition of cancer cell proliferation in vitro by fruit and berry extracts and correlations with antioxidant levels.** Olsson ME, Gustavsson KE, Andersson S, Nilsson A, Duan RD. Department of Crop Science, Swedish University of Agricultural Sciences Alnarp, Sweden.

Abstract. The effects of 10 different extracts of fruits and berries on cell proliferation of colon cancer cells HT29 and breast cancer cells MCF-7 were investigated. The fruits and berries used were rosehips, blueberries, black currant, black chokeberries, apple, sea buckthorn, plum, lingonberries, cherries, and raspberries. The extracts decreased the proliferation of both colon cancer cells HT29 and breast cancer cells MCF-7, and the effect was concentration dependent. The inhibition effect for the highest concentration of the extracts varied 2-3-fold among the species, and it was in the ranges of 46-74% (average = 62%) for the HT29 cells and 24-68% (average = 52%) for the MCF-7 cells. There were great differences in the content of the analyzed antioxidants in the extracts. The level of the vitamin C content varied almost 100-fold, and the content of total carotenoids varied almost 150-fold among the species. Also in the composition and content of flavonols, hydroxycinnamic acids, anthocyanins, and phenolics were found great differences among the 10 species. *The inhibition of cancer cell proliferation seen in these experiments correlated with levels of some carotenoids and with vitamin C levels, present at levels that can be found in human tissues.*

Interpretation. This valuable in vitro study showed that carotenoids from berries could inhibit activity of colon cancer cells at concentrations correlating with carotenoid levels in humans. Although wolfberries were not included in the analysis, their high carotenoid content indicates that wolfberries would be an excellent dietary source to provide this anti-cancer effect in vivo.

Oxygen Radical Absorbance Capacity, ORAC

Oxidative stress is associated with increased risk of developing several diseases, including cancer, cardiovascular and inflammatory disorders, neuronal degeneration (such as Alzheimer's and Parkinson's disease) and the general deterioration that occurs with aging.

Oxidative stress results from the activities of reactive oxygen species (ROS) that damage cell elements such as proteins, lipids, membranes and DNA. ROS evolve from normal body functions that are usually in balance during health.

However, when balancing mechanisms are ineffective—perhaps because of a diet poor in antioxidant foods—ROS disperse randomly in a concentration gradient from their point of formation, so may do considerable cellular damage within cells and to nearby cells where they are formed, contributing to disease and aging.

As we have heard in public news on diets, intake of a variety of fruits and vegetables is the best solution for ingesting antioxidant compounds from plants, or "phytochemicals" as discussed in Chapter 2. Vitamins A, C and E, carotenoids, phenolics and select minerals like zinc, manganese and selenium are mentioned as common antioxidant nutrients available from dietary sources.

In a review of antioxidant phytochemicals, Lee and coworkers described laboratory measurements of oxygen radical activity and its quenching specifically by carotenoids (see References). They stated that *"carotenoids are the most efficient singlet oxygen quencher in biological systems."* An interesting result from laboratory measurements of ORAC would be to compare the strength of primarily carotenoid foods with those that have phenolics as their main antioxidant quality. We're not aware that such a comparison is available.

We also learned above that isolating these antioxidant phytochemcials individually and using them as separate supplements have not always produced the most successful results in clinical trials on large numbers of people. In other words, an antioxidant nutrient by itself is not assured to provide the desired nutritional benefit—eating foods with all of the antioxidants contained—as indicated by the term "phytonutrient synergy"—would give the greatest dietary benefit.

Recently, a database of ORAC values was published by members of the US Department of Agriculture (References, Wu et al., 2004, see Chapter 12) who had devised test tube measurements of ORAC that would allow comparison of antioxidant qualities among different foods. The test includes both lipid-favoring ("lipophilic" as carotenoids would have) and water-favoring ("hydrophilic" as phenolic agents would have) antioxidant nutrients to be measured in the same plant, resulting in an added value of these two components to give "total ORAC".

This ORAC test will likely gain in public acceptance over coming years as it will allow relationships for comparing antioxidant values on food labels, choosing high ORAC foods selectively and relating antioxidant capacity to disease incidence. For example, already there has been established an inverse correlation between antioxidant intake and incidence of some cancers, e.g., above publications 30-31.

Preliminary analyses of ORAC for wolfberries have been posted on the web by Young Living for background on Berry Young Juice and Ningxia Red juice (see web reference in Chapter 12).

The results show a value of 30,000 micromoles of Trolox equivalents (total ORAC units) per 100 grams compared to about 9260 for wild blueberries and 2640 for spinach (data from Wu et al., 2004; no data available for papaya). If confirmed, such a high ORAC for wolfberries would place it as the highest ranking fruit and among the strongest antioxidant foods known. Interestingly, herbs such as cloves and cinnamon have even 10x higher ORAC values (dried material, Wu et al., 2004) than wolfberries.

Hopefully, future research will further examine this apparently exceptional antioxidant strength of wolfberries, including the division of ORAC components between lipid-soluble carotenoids and water-soluble phenolics.

What health conditions require special emphasis on carotenoids and their potential antioxidant benefit against diseases? The website, World's Healthiest Foods (Chapter 12 references), offers this list

- Age-related macular degeneration
- Acquired Immunodeficiency Syndrome (AIDS)
- Angina pectoris
- Asthma
- Cataracts
- Cervical dysplasia
- Vaginal candidiasis
- Chlamydial infection
- Heart disease
- Male and female infertility
- Osteoarthritis
- Photosensitivity
- Pneumonia
- Rheumatoid arthritis
- Cervical cancer
- Lung cancer
- Laryngeal cancer
- Skin cancer
- Prostate cancer

疾病

CHAPTER 6
Wolfberry Phytochemicals And Disease Research:
Implied Health Benefits

Beginning in Chapter 3 with presentation of wolfberry's multiple nutrients, we started to assemble a nutrition-based profile about wolfberry's implicated health benefits. In Chapters 4 and 5 on wolfberry polysaccharides and carotenoids, respectively, we zeroed in on signature nutrients that have received the most scientific validation.

Here in this chapter, we extend this analysis of nutrition-health relationships by presenting summaries of PubMed citations on as many published works about wolfberries as available at the time of this writing (September 2005). Several novel phytochemicals of potential health interest emerge.

As typical consumers, we are particularly focused on how consumption of a reputed health food like wolfberries may affect our overall health and offset risk or progression of diseases. Much of this preliminary understanding is both inferred and premature to conclude that such benefits actually exist, but is nevertheless useful to consider the available studies and summarize categories of health benefits.

We may have made errors in selecting material or interpreting results from the literature given below. Most literature is only in abstract form mainly from Chinese publications translated into English, so there are limitations possibly in the amount of information and in its translation. We selectively edited each abstract to give the clearest possible view for the general consumer. In not all cases, however, did we eliminate scientific terminology in the abstracts as we wanted to retain interest for scientists reading this book.

More fascinating details about wolfberries result, giving broad based nutrition information for diets, traditional medicine and health benefits. Some of these lessons have been handed down in China through centuries of legends about wolfberries.

Before examining relationships between wolfberry phytochemicals and health benefits, it's important to gain a view of the most definitive type of clinical study that would allow health claims about nutrients or drugs—clinical trials (see also Chapter 2).

Clinical Trials and Food Science Standards

Clinical trials are carefully controlled research studies that measure how well a new drug, treatment or undefined nutrient performs compared to a "standard treatment" currently available. In first-world countries, trials are required by law to prove efficacy and safety before a new drug can be approved for market. In the US, the Food & Drug Administration (FDA) or any country's regulatory agency for drugs or foods (e.g., European Medicines Evaluation Agency, EMEA or Health Canada) is the body overseeing design, analysis and conclusions of clinical trials.

Particularly for natural products like berries and their potential nutritional benefits for health and disease prevention, Health Canada's Natural Products Directorate, as an example, has been redesigned to accommodate and encourage clinical research projects (Reference in Chapter 2, see Chapter 12). As the natural products industry grows worldwide, more regulatory authorities like the FDA and EMEA will devote specific attention to guidelines on clinical research of foods and nutrients.

Clinical trials are valuable for determining the *best* conditions of using nutrients as supplements or dietary replacements for given health or disease conditions, and are crucial for identifying potential side effects or adverse reactions.

As there are systematic steps in a formal multiyear clinical trial, called phases 1 through 4, the burden of time and costs for such intensive research falls on the sponsoring company, often costing millions (or tens of millions) of dollars for additional expenses to bring the tested agent into approval status. Not all food and nutrient companies (in fact, few companies?) can afford these expensive regulatory obligations.

Perhaps they should not have to fulfill them. After all, functional foods and nutritional supplements are products chosen independently by consumers over regular foods because such foods are assumed to furnish a health benefit or appeal to more subjective sensory qualities like taste and aroma.

Nutrient research does not require the same rigor for satisfying safety as would apply to a completely novel drug proposed for use in patients, yet most countries still frame nutrient clinical trials in the testing model for drugs. One can readily see the problems confronting clinical trial design for nutrients by considering potential interactions that must be accounted for in the design of the study between dietary habits, similar foods, age, gender, genetic factors, illness and drugs prescribed for specific medical conditions.

This preamble applies to all so-called "functional" foods as wolfberries are, i.e., multinutrient food sources that may benefit human health via individual or many nutrients acting in synergy. And this interaction occurs in the presence of other foods eaten and other factors influencing health or disease.

We must therefore be very cautious about assigning health benefits from consumption of one food source like wolfberries unless appropriate isolation of the beneficial nutrient has been incorporated into a clinical trial—virtually an impossible task in food science.

As one intention of this book is to present interpretations of health benefits wolfberries may provide, we want to gather those publications now in this chapter and help establish a basis for judging wolfberry's nutrients in the context of health and disease prevention, as legend has offered over centuries.

Thus, we hope that a modest amount of skepticism is now instilled in the reader so that not all health claims of wolfberries are accepted outright. More research is needed to get us beyond this skepticism into the realm of scientific validation, fact and consumer acceptance.

To summarize what is included in this chapter, we present study claims (where applicable), abstracts and synopses of research on some of the chemical isolation studies on wolfberries, often the first step toward defining a specific health benefit. Following then are categories of research on organ systems and diseases grouped broadly into potential major health effects and diseases—cardiovascular system, aging, metabolic processes, and inflammatory disorders. Abstract titles enclosed in brackets [like this] indicate that the original publication was in Chinese.

Phyto-and Biochemistry

This section addresses plant ("phyto") and biochemical findings that underlie physiological actions within the body. The science mainly addresses individual chemicals with possible health applications, but requires further validation studies and testing for specific organ or health effects.

There is no special order of the following applications of wolfberry phytochemicals. Collectively, however, the information displays a diversity of interesting compounds in wolfberries pointing toward possible commercial applications of using this berry as a whole food or for its specific extracts.

1. **Study Claim.** The novel wolfberry chemical, monomenthyl succinate, having menthol-like qualities, may be extracted as an additive for toothpastes and mouth rinses.

Publication. J. Agric Food Chem. 2004 Jun 2;52(11):3536-41. **Identification of monomenthyl succinate, monomenthyl glutarate, and dimenthyl glutarate in nature by high performance liquid chromatography-tandem mass spectrometry.** Hiserodt RD, Adedeji J, John TV, Dewis ML. International Flavors & Fragrances Inc, Research and Development, Union Beach, NJ, USA.

Abstract. Menthol, menthone, and other natural compounds provide a cooling effect and a minty flavor and have found wide application in chewing gum and oral care products. Monomenthyl succinate, monomenthyl glutarate, and dimenthyl glutarate provide a cooling effect without the burning sensation associated with menthol. Additionally, because they do not have a distinct flavor, they can be used in applications other than mint flavors. Because these menthyl esters have not been reported in nature, we undertook to identify a natural source for these cooling compounds. Using high performance liquid chromatography and mass spectrometry, monomenthyl succinate was identified in Lycium barbarum and Mentha piperita, and monomenthyl glutarate and dimenthyl glutarate were identified in Litchi chinesis. The identifications were based on the correlation of mass spectrometric and chromatographic data for the menthyl esters.

Synopsis. Monomenthyl succinate is a plant constituent with mouth-or skin-cooling effects, no burning sensation and no after-taste. This substance is present in wolfberries, indicating a useful extraction that could be made for flavoring foods, medicines, toothpastes, skin creams, etc.

2. Study Claim. Pyrrole extracts from wolfberries resemble the antioxidant flavanone, silybin, and have protective effects on liver cells.

Publication. Bioorg Med Chem Lett. 2003 Jan 6;13(1):79-81. **Hepatoprotective pyrrole derivatives of Lycium chinense fruits.** Chin YW, Lim SW, Kim SH, Shin DY, Suh YG, Kim YB, Kim YC, Kim J. College of Pharmacy and Research Institute of Pharmaceutical Science, Seoul National University, South Korea.

Abstract. As a part of our search for hepatoprotective compounds from Lycium chinense fruits, three new pyrrole derivatives, 1-3, were isolated. These compounds and a 4th related synthetic methylated compound were evaluated for their biological activity and structure-activity relationship. Compounds 1 and 2 showed hepatoprotective effects comparable to silybin.

Synopsis. 4 new compounds were isolated from wolfberries. One of them, a pyrrole with similarities to silybin, is a naturally occurring flavanone (polyphenol) having antioxidant functions. Silybin (silymarin or silibinin from milk thistle) has been identified with anti-cancer effects and protection of liver cells from toxicity in laboratory models.

3. Publication. Arch Pharm Res. 2002 Aug;25(4):433-7. **A new phenolic amide from Lycium chinense Miller.** Han SH, Lee HH, Lee IS, Moon YH, Woo ER. College of Pharmacy, Chosun University, Kwang-ju, Korea.

Abstract. A new phenolic amide, dihydro-N-caffeoyltyramine (1) was isolated from the root bark of Lycium chinense Miller, along with known compounds, trans-N-caffeoyltyramine (2), cis-N-caffeoyltyramine (3), and lyoniresinol 3-alpha-O-beta-D-glucopyranoside (4). Their structures were determined by spectroscopic analysis. A superoxide scavenging assay revealed that three phenolic amides showed potent antioxidative activity.

4. Publication. Zhongguo Zhong Yao Za Zhi. 2001 May;26(5):323-4. **[Studies on chemical constituents in fruit of Lycium barbarum L.]** [Article in Chinese] Xie C, Xu LZ, Li XM, Li KM, Zhao BH, Yang SL. Institute of Medicinal Plant Development, Chinese Academy of Medical Sciences, Peking Union Medical College, Beijing, China.

Abstract. Objective: To study the chemical constituents in the fruit of Lycium barbarum. Method: The chemical constituents were isolated by column chromatography and identified by spectral data. Result: The compounds obtained were identified as scopoletin (I), beta-sitosterol (II), p-coumaric acid (III), glucose (IV), daucosterol (V) and betaine (VI). Conclusion: Compounds III, IV and V were isolated from Lycium barbarum for the first time.

Synopsis. This extraction study showed the presence of several interesting compounds from wolfberry fruit. **p-Coumaric acid**, an antioxidant phenolic acid, was identified for the first time. This is a valuable result, indicating that wolfberry may contain 2 significant classes of antioxidant phytochemicals—carotenoids, as discussed in Chapter 5, and phenolics, briefly covered in Chapters 2 and 3. **Scopoletin** is also a member of the coumarin chemical family (polyphenolic antioxidants) that inhibits the enzyme degrading acetylcholine, a transmitter in the nervous system. Consequently, scopoletin would prolong acetylcholine's activity. It also suppresses inflammatory enzymes, so may be useful as an anti-inflammatory agent.

Beta-sitosterol is a plant sterol or phytosterol, a class of compounds known to inhibit cholesterol uptake (Chapter 3) and so can reduce circulating blood levels of cholesterol. Beta-sitosterol has also been shown to suppress growth of breast cancer cells in vitro.

p-Coumaric acid, belonging to the phenolic class of antioxidants found in red grapes and wine, has been shown to upregulate the enzyme that synthesizes nitric oxide (nitric oxide synthase), the endothelium-resident relaxing factor that dilates small arteries and arterioles. This finding indicates that p-coumaric acid participates in regulation of local blood flow in organs.

Daucosterol is related to sitosterol in the family of phytosterols (Chapter 3), compounds that have anti-cholesterol and anti-platelet (or anti-clotting) mechanisms.

Lastly, as a methyl donor, **betaine** has several complex effects in the body, including lowering of homocysteine levels in cardiovascular and liver disease, and fat weight gain. Betaine has also been attributed with anti-fatigue properties. Chinese research has stated that wolfberries contain approximately 1 mg of betaine per gram of dried fruit.

5. **Publication.** J Chromatogr A. 1999 Oct 1;857(1-2):331-5. **Determination of betaine in Lycium chinense fruits by liquid**

chromatography-electrospray ionization mass spectrometry. Shin YG, Cho KH, Kim JM, Park MK, Park JH. College of Pharmacy, Seoul National University, South Korea.

Abstract. A rapid and sensitive high-performance liquid chromatography and mass spectrometric method was developed for the determination of betaine in wolfberry fruit.

6. **Study Claim.** The study focuses on phytochemicals from wolfberry fruit that affect mucin release (or lubricating mechanisms) in airway diseases. The chemicals betaine and hesperidin increased mucin activity and so wolfberry consumption may have beneficial effects in respiratory disorders.

Publication. Phytother Res. 2004 Apr;18(4):301-5. **Effects of betaine, coumarin and flavonoids on mucin release from cultured hamster tracheal surface epithelial cells.** Lee CJ, Lee JH, Seok JH, Hur GM, Park Js J, Bae S, Lim JH, Park YC. Department of Pharmacology, College of Medicine, Chungnam National University, Daejeon, Korea.

Abstract. Betaine, coumarin, hesperidin and kaempferol are the components derived from Lycium chinense, Angelicae decursiva, Poncirus trifoliata and Polygonatum odoratum, respectively. These plants have been used for the treatment of respiratory diseases in oriental medicine and their respective components were reported to have various biological effects. In this study, the authors investigated whether these natural products affect mucin release from cultured hamster tracheal surface epithelial cells and compared the possible activities of these agents with the inhibitory action on mucin release by poly-L-lysine and the stimulatory action by adenosine triphosphate. The results were as follows: (i) Coumarin and kaempferol did not affect mucin release significantly; (ii) Betaine and hesperidin increased mucin release at the highest concentration; (iii) Poly-L-lysine inhibited and adenosine triphosphate increased mucin release. The authors conclude that betaine and hesperidin can increase mucin release by directly acting on airway mucin-secreting cells and suggest these agents be further studied for the possible use as mild expectorants during the treatment of chronic airway diseases.

Synopsis. We discussed before the methyl donor, betaine, found in wolfberries. Having a variety of roles, betaine is involved in cardiovascular, liver and fat metabolism. It may be an anti-fatigue agent via mechanisms poorly understood. In this study, wolfberry betaine is proposed as an airway mucin stimulant or alternatively, as an expectorant potentially valuable in cold and cough remedies. Chronic respiratory disorders, such as asthma and obstructive pulmonary disease, may also be aided by wolfberry betaine.

7. Publication. Zhongguo Zhong Yao Za Zhi. 1995 May;20(5):303-4. **[Protective action of Lycium barbarum L. (LbL) and betaine on lipid peroxidation of erythrocyte membrane induced by hydrogen peroxide]** [Article in Chinese] Ren B, Ma Y, Shen Y, Gao B. Faculty of Preventive Medicine, Ningxia Medical College, Yinchuan, China.

Abstract. Hydrogen peroxide was used to induce lipid peroxidation of red blood cell membranes in rats to observe the protective action of different ingredients of wolfberry preparations, including polysaccharides, and betaine on the membrane. The result shows these ingredients can inhibit the lipid peroxidation of red cell membranes in the following order of antioxidizing power: Fructus Lycii.LbL.dry(FL/LbL.dry) > Polysaccharide FL/LbL > Residue FL/LbL > betaine.

Synopsis. This study reveals possible antioxidant properties of betaine and polysaccharides from wolfberries in isolated red blood cell membranes from rats. Identity of the wolfberry nutrients and specific polysaccharide(s) involved in preventing the oxidation of the blood cell membranes was not provided.

8. Publication. Eur J Biochem. 1997 Sep 1;248(2):296-303. **Specific alpha-galactosidase inhibitors, N-methylcalystegines-structure/ activity relationships of calystegines from Lycium chinense.** Asano N, Kato A, Miyauchi M, Kizu H, Tomimori T, Matsui K, Nash RJ, Molyneux RJ. Faculty of Pharmaceutical Sciences, Hokuriku University, Kanazawa, Japan.

Abstract. An examination of the roots of Lycium chinense has resulted in the discovery of 14 calystegines. L. chinense also had two polyhydroxytropanes. 1-Beta-amino-3-beta, 4-beta, 5-alpha-trihydroxycycloheptane was also present in L. chinense and may be a biosynthetic precursor of the calystegines that occur in this plant. Since this compound is a very specific inhibitor of alpha-galactosidase and inhibits rat liver lysosomal alpha-galactosidase, it may provide a useful experimental model for the lysosomal storage disorder, Fabry's disease.

Synopsis. Calystegines are alkaloid compounds (substances containing nitrogen) characteristic of the extensive family of plants to which wolfberries belong—Solanaceae (see Chapter 8). This study was done on wolfberry root extracts. Calystegines inhibit an enzyme called alpha-galactosidase that is absent in Fabry's disease, a lysosome storage disorder. To understand this disease better, an experimental model may be created in animals treated with wolfberry calystegines.

9. **Publication.** Se Pu. 1997 Jan;15(1):54-6. [**Determination of taurine in Lycium barbarum L. by high performance liquid chromatography with OPA-urea pre-column derivatization**] [Article in Chinese] Xie H, Zhang S. Department of Food Science and Technology, Huazhong Agricultural University, Wuhan, China.

Abstract. Dried Lycium barbarum L. was prepared for high performance liquid chromatographic separation. Taurine was determined quantitatively.

Synopsis. Taurine is a nonessential amino acid, meaning that it is synthesized from other amino acids in plants or in the liver of mammals; it does not have to be obtained directly through the diet.

Taurine is synthesized from the essential amino acid methionine. It works as a membrane amino acid that helps the cell to retain potassium. In the central nervous system of mammals, taurine facilitates activity of inhibitory neurotransimitters, i.e., transmitter chemicals that turn off neuronal activity. In studies on mice, taurine has been shown to help retain memory. Taurine is also necessary for management of potassium levels in tissues such as the heart where potassium has delicate roles in cellular excitability.

10. **Publication.** J Agric Food Chem. 2001 Jun;49(6):3101-5. **Alpha-tocopherol content in 62 edible tropical plants.** Ching LS, Mohamed S. Faculty of Food Science and Biotechnology, University Putra Malaysia, Serdang Selangor, Malaysia.

Abstract. Alpha-tocopherol (Vitamin E) was determined by HPLC. All the plants tested showed differences in their alpha-tocopherol content. The highest alpha-tocopherol content was in Sauropus androgynus leaves (426.8 mg/kg edible portion), followed by Citrus hystrix leaves (398.3 mg/kg), Calamus scipronum (193.8 mg/kg), starfruit leaves Averrhoa belimbi (168.3 mg/kg), red pepper Capsicum annum (155.4 mg/kg), local celery Apium graveolens (136.4 mg/kg), sweet potato shoots Ipomoea batatas (130.1 mg/kg), Pandanus odorus (131.5 mg/kg), Oenanthe javanica (146.8 mg/kg), black tea Camelia chinensis (183.3 mg/kg), **papaya** Carica papaya shoots (111.3 mg/kg) and **wolfberry leaves** Lycium chinense (94.4 mg/kg).

Synopsis. Vitamin E is not a common nutrient of berry fruit and indeed this study did not reveal it in wolfberries. Vitamin E was found, however, in wolfberry leaves.

11. **Publication.** Wei Sheng Yan Jiu. 1999 Mar 30;28(2):115-6. [**The protective effects of total flavonoids from Lycium barbarum L. on lipid peroxidation of liver mitochondria and red blood cells in rats**] [Article in Chinese] Huang Y, Lu J, Shen Y, Lu J. Dept. of Nutrition and Food Hygiene, Faculty of Preventive Medicine, Ningxia Medical College, Yinchuan, China.

Abstract. The protective effects of total flavonoids from Lycium barbarum L. on lipid peroxidation in mitochondria and red blood cells induced by oxygen radicals were investigated. The mitochondria lipid peroxidation (measured as malondialdehyde) was significantly inhibited by wolfberry flavonoids with a dose-response relationship.

Synopsis. Unidentified wolfberry flavonoids protected mitochondria and red blood cells from lipid peroxidation, a process of oxidative damage to cell membranes. Unfortunately, there is insufficient information in this abstract to judge the importance of this finding and to identify specific flavonoids present in wolfberries.

As emphasized in this book, wolfberry's carotenoids likely contribute the most powerful antioxidant qualities of the fruit. However, if flavonoids were also present in sufficient quantities, a dual action of these two antioxidant classes may provide unusually strong antioxidant benefit from wolfberry consumption. This would represent a nutrient synergy so well recognized from eating whole foods. More research is clearly needed on this valuable topic.

Wolfberry Health and Disease Properties

Cardiovascular System

12. **Publication.** Sheng Li Xue Bao. 1998 Jun;50(3):309-14. [**The effect of lycium barbarum polysaccharide on vascular tension in two-kidney, one clip model of hypertension**] [Article in Chinese] Jia YX, Dong JW, Wu XX, Ma TM, Shi AY. Department of Pathophysiology, Beijing Medical University, Beijing, China.

Abstract. The effects of lycium barbarum polysaccharide (LBP) on endothelial and vascular functions in the two-kidney, one clip model of hypertension were observed. The results showed that the increase of blood pressure in hypertension rats could be prevented significantly by treatment with 10% LBP. In isolated aortic rings of LBP-treated rats, the contraction of phenylephrine (PE) was reduced. Removal of the endothelium abolished the difference of PE-induced vasoconstriction among groups, indicating the response derives from the endothelial cells. In vitro incubation of aortic rings from LBP-treated rats with methylene blue or N-nitro-L-arginine methyl ester (L-NAME) increased the magnitude of PE-induced contractions. Meanwhile the response to acetylcholine (ACh) was significantly increased in LBP-treated rats, but the response to nitroprusside had no significant difference among groups. Pretreatment with L-arginine partially restored ACh-induced relaxation in hypertensive rats, but there was no such effect in LBP-treated rats. The results suggest that the role of LBP in decreasing vasoconstriction to PE may be mediated by increase of the effects or/and production of endothelium-derived relaxation factor (EDRF). Increased formation of EDRF from LBP may in turn increase the substrate of EDRF, i.e., formation of nitric oxide.

Synopsis. This interesting and thorough study examined the effects of wolfberry polysaccharides on vascular responses in rats with experimental hypertension. The results reported are that wolfberry polysaccharides could attenuate the development of high blood pressure and afforded vascular segments improved ability to relax (interpreted as dilation of the intact blood vessel).

Mechanisms involving acetylcholine and formation of the endothelium-derived relaxing factor (nitric oxide from arginine) appear to be important for these effects. Endothelial cells form the inner layer of arteries, arterioles, venules and veins, and are the main component of the smallest blood vessels, capillaries.

In the intact healthy animal or human, the results infer that wolfberry polysaccharides impart a beneficial effect for regulating normal blood pressure and counteracting high blood pressure via a pathway involving the vascular endothelial cells that form nitric oxide, the endothelium-derived relaxing factor.

Anti-Apoptosis, Anti-Aging, Metabolic Properties

13. **Publication.** J Ethnopharmacol. 1993 Mar;38(2-3):167-75.

Immunological aspects of Chinese medicinal plants as antiaging drugs. Xiao PG, Xing ST, Wang LW. Institute of Medicinal Plant Development, Chinese Academy of Medical Sciences, Beijing, China.

Abstract. The development of a predominantly geriatric community worldwide has become an inevitable fact. Anti-aging agents could be, in a certain sense, attentive to the well-being of the aged. There are quite a lot of medicinal plants and prescriptions recorded in Chinese medical literatures aimed at the well-being of the aged as well as the prevention of diseases and prolongation of life-span. By means of modern scientific research, a strategy towards anti-aging drugs is presented in this paper. One of the effective routes is to select the candidates based on their ethnopharmacological usages, followed by immunological investigation in connection with other anti-aging experimentation. Chinese medicinal plants used as (or related to) anti-aging agents are presented. Specifically, five Chinese traditional drugs, Herba Epimedii, **Fructus Lycii**, Radix Polygoni multiflori, Radix Cynanchi auriculati and **Ganoderma** along with a composite prescription 'American Ginseng Royal Jelly' are selected as representatives. The prospect of research and development of anti-aging drugs based on natural origin is also discussed.

Synopsis. This 1993 report acknowledged both wolfberries and Ganoderma mushrooms as traditional Chinese "drugs" possibly beneficial as anti-aging foods. Unfortunately, the abstract lacks information to provide scientific evidence for how these food sources could establish anti-aging benefits.

14. **Publication.** Zhong Yao Cai. 1999 May;22(5):250-1. [The regulation of Lycium barbarum on apoptosis of rat spleen in vitro] [Article in Chinese] Lu X, Xian X, Lu W, Wu X, Gu H. Guangdong College of Pharmacy, Guangzhou, China.

Abstract. The regulation of Lycium barbarum (LB) on apoptosis of rat spleen induced by hydrocortisone (HYD) was studied. LB could inhibit the apoptosis induced by HYD and the inhibition was dose dependent.

Synopsis. Apoptosis ("eh-poe-toe-sis"), the natural mechanism of cells dying, may be a major mechanism of age-related decline of body functions. Wolfberry preparations inhibited apoptosis in this study. The results are insufficient to judge the work but indicate a possible mechanism regulating cell function and apoptosis by wolfberry constituents.

15. **Publication.** Biomed Environ Sci. 2003 Sep;16(3):267-75. **Inhibiting effects of Achyranthes bidentata polysaccharide and Lycium barbarum polysaccharide on nonenzyme glycation in D-galactose induced mouse aging model.** Deng HB, Cui DP, Jiang JM, Feng YC, Cai NS, Li DD. Institute of Medicinal Biotechnology, Chinese Academy of Medical Sciences, Peking Union Medical College, Beijing, China.

Abstract. Objective: To investigate the inhibiting effects and mechanism of achyranthes bidentata polysaccharide (ABP) and lycium barbarum polysaccharide (LBP) on nonenzyme glycation in D-galactose induced mouse aging model. Results: Decreased levels of spontaneous motor activity in D-galactose mouse aging model were detected after treatment with ABP or LBP, while lymphocyte proliferation and IL-2 activity, learning and memory abilities, SOD activity of erythrocytes, were enhanced.

Synopsis. In this mouse model of aging, an unnamed wolfberry polysaccharide reduced the spontaneous motor activity of mice and increased lymphocyte levels, interleukin-2 levels, memory, and activity of the antioxidant enzyme, superoxide dismutase. The authors conclude the results showed an anti-aging effect in the mice. Although rudimentary, this research provides a basis for further examination of several potentially interesting effects of wolfberries on immune responsiveness, physical activity, memory and cognition, and antioxidant mechanisms.

16. **Publication.** Wei Sheng Yan Jiu. 2002 Feb;31(1):30-1. **[Effect of lycium barbarum L on defending free radicals caused by hypoxia in mice]** [Article in Chinese] Li G, Yang J, Ren B, Wang Z. Faculty of Preventive Medicine, Ningxia Medicine College, Yinchuan, China.

Abstract. The effect of Lycium Barbarum L. (LB) on the free radical defending system during hypoxia was tested. Fifty-six mice were divided into 3 groups. Experimental mice were fed with LB and the control mice were fed with distilled water by tube feeding for 16 days. Animals were put into each enclosed bottle for testing the effect of hypoxia (low air oxygen levels). The results showed that LB treatment could not prolong the survival time, but increased activities of superoxide dismutase, catalase and total anti-oxidative capacity as compared with the control group. The study indicated that LB might have a protective effect on free radical injury caused by hypoxia.

Synopsis. Low oxygen levels in air ("hypoxia") are used in this study to challenge antioxidant responses of mice provided either with wolfberries in their diet or with only normal food and water (control group). Mice fed with wolfberries had raised levels of 2 antioxidant enzymes and total antioxidant capacity, indicating that some constituent of the berry afforded mice with these protective nutrients.

Based on our analyses above, we can speculate that the carotenoids—beta-carotene, zeaxanthin and cryptoxanthin—and antioxidant vitamins and minerals—vitamins A, C and E and minerals zinc, magnesium, manganese, copper and selenium—have such a role.

17. **Publication.** Ann Pharmacother. 2001 Oct;35(10):1199-201. **Possible interaction between warfarin and Lycium barbarum L.** Lam AY, Elmer GW, Mohutsky MA., Department of Pharmacy, University of Washington, Seattle, USA.

Abstract. Objective: To describe a patient who was stabilized on warfarin and developed an elevated international normalized ratio (INR) after drinking a concentrated Chinese herbal tea made from wolfberries. An elevated INR of 4.1 was observed in a 61-year-old Chinese woman, previously stabilized on anticoagulation therapy (INR 2-3). With no changes in her other medications or lifestyle, a review of her dietary habits revealed four days of drinking a concentrated Chinese herbal tea made from Lycium barbarum L. fruits (3-4 glasses daily) prior to her clinic visit. Warfarin was withheld for one day and then resumed at a lower weekly dose. She discontinued the tea, while maintaining consistency with medications and dietary habits. A follow-up INR seven days later was 2.4, and seven subsequent INR values were in the 2.0-2.5 range. Lycium barbarum L. (wolfberry) is a commonly used Chinese herb considered to have a tonic effect on various organs. Any impact of an herbal product on the metabolism of S-warfarin, the enantiomer responsible for most of the anticoagulant activity, could alter INR values. An herbal-drug interaction was suspected in this case. In vitro evaluation showed inhibition of S-warfarin metabolism by the tea of L. barbarum L. Conclusion: There is a potential herbal-drug interaction between warfarin and wolfberry based on an increased INR value noted with concurrent use. Thus, combination of L. barbarum L. and warfarin should be avoided. Vigilance is needed with other herbal combinations taken with drugs of narrow therapeutic indices.

Synopsis. In this often-cited study, wolfberry consumption in the form of tea *by one patient* appeared to increase the blood-thinning actions of warfarin (coumadin), a drug commonly used orally as an anti-coagulant or "blood-thinner" after heart attack or blood clots. Only one patient was studied, giving question about how such an effect would occur across many users. The authors concluded that metabolism of the enzyme degrading warfarin may be affected by wolfberry nutrients, and so patients taking this drug for anti-coagulation should avoid wolfberry consumption (which would further elevate the effects of warfarin).

In our discussion in Chapter 4 of terpenes in Ganoderma mushrooms, we saw that a blood-thinning effect may occur through inhibition of thromboxane A, the enzyme responsible for attenuating platelet aggregation. Inferring, this would mean that wolfberry terpenes (beta-carotene may be one) could inhibit thromboxane A, leading to less platelet aggregation (reduced clotting ability) and a greater anti-coagulant effect than from just warfarin alone. Such an effect, however, needs a more complete clinical investigation to allow this conclusion.

18. Publication. Zhong Yao Cai. 2002 Sep;25(9):649-51. [The protective effects of Lycium barbarum polysaccharide on alloxan-induced isolated islet cells damage in rats] [Article in Chinese] Xu M, Zhang H, Wang Y. School of Life Science, East China Normal University, Shanghai, China.

Abstract. Objective: To study the effects of Lycium barbarum polysaccharide (LBP) on alloxan-induced isolated islet cells damage in rats. Isolated islet cells from rats were cultured in vitro. Superoxide dismutase (SOD) activity and malondialdehyde (MDA) content in rat islet cells incubated with alloxan or alloxan combined LBP were measured. Alloxan induced a significant decrease in SOD activity and an increase in MDA production, which were inhibited by LBP. Conclusion: LBP had protective effects on alloxan-induced isolated rat islet cell damage.

Synopsis. This study used cells isolated from the pancreas of rats ("islet cells") as a model of diabetes mellitus. The chemical alloxan, a toxin to islet cells, was applied to create oxidative stress, with 2 chemicals assessed to gauge the extent of injury. SOD is an antioxidant enzyme and MDA is a product of oxidation. Wolfberry polysaccharide (LBP) inhibited both effects of alloxan so demonstrated antioxidant protection.

19. Publication. J Ethnopharmacol. 2002 Oct;82(2-3):169-75.

Protective effect of Fructus Lycii polysaccharides against time and hyperthermia-induced damage in cultured seminiferous epithelium. Wang Y, Zhao H, Sheng X, Gambino PE, Costello B, Bojanowski K. Department of Histology and Embryology, Ningxia Medical College, Yinchuan, China.

Abstract. Lycium barbarum L. (Solanaceae) is a Chinese medicinal plant whose fruits (Fructus Lycii) are used by Chinese physicians for treatment of infertility. However, the active ingredients and the mechanism of action underlying Lycium's fertility-facilitating effects remain unknown. Here we report that Fructus Lycii polysaccharides (FLPS) inhibit time—and hyperthermia-induced structural damage in murine seminiferous epithelium in vitro. Moreover, we found that FLPS delayed apoptosis in this system, both at normothermic and hyperthermic culture conditions. Oxidative stress was reported to be a major cause of structural degradation and apoptosis in hyperthermic testes, and thus the protective effect of FLPS could implicate an antioxidant mechanism of action. To test this hypothesis we assayed the effect of FLPS on ultraviolet light-induced lipid peroxidation, and cytochrome c reduction by free radicals. We found that FLPS is a potent inhibitor of both of these reactions. Together, these results demonstrate the protective effect of FLPS on time—and hyperthermia-induced testicular degeneration in vitro, indicate the potential mechanism of action for this protective effect, and provide a scientific basis for the traditional use of this plant.

Synopsis. This study was performed to model the effect of wolfberries on testicular cells (seminiferous epithelium, or semen-producing cells) simulating the fertility benefits wolfberry reportedly has by legend and TCM practice. We do not learn how polysaccharides were isolated or which one(s) were used in this research. Wolfberry polysaccharides reduced the effects of high temperature and ultraviolet light (an antioxidant model) on apoptosis and free radical damage of mouse testicular cells in vitro. Although it's a leap to say these findings support the enhanced fertility claims attributed by legend to eating wolfberries, they provide in vitro support for the antioxidant role of polysaccharides.

20. **Publication.** Exp Gerontol. 2005 Aug-Sep;40(8-9):716-27. **Neuroprotective effects of anti-aging oriental medicine Lycium barbarum against beta-amyloid peptide neurotoxicity.** Yu MS, Leung SK, Lai SW, Che CM, Zee SY, So KF, Yuen WH, Chang RC,

Laboratory of Neurodegenerative Diseases, Department of Anatomy, University of Hong Kong, Hong Kong.

Abstract. As aged populations dramatically increase in these decades, efforts should be made on the intervention for curing age-associated neurodegenerative diseases such as Alzheimer's disease (AD). Natural plant extracts of Lycium barbarum (LB) are thought to exhibit anti-aging effects. The authors hypothesized that LB exhibits neuroprotective effects against toxins in aging-related neurodegenerative diseases. The authors aimed to investigate whether extracts from LB have neuroprotective effects against toxicity of fibrillar amyloid-beta(1-42) and amyloid-beta(25-35) fragments. Primary rat cortical neurons exposed to amyloid-beta peptides resulted in apoptosis and necrosis. Pre-treatment with LB extract significantly reduced the release of lactate dehydrogenase (LDH). In addition, LB attenuated amyloid-beta peptide-activated caspases-3-like activity. The extract elicited a typical dose-dependent neuroprotective effect in vitro. The authors further examined underlying mechanisms of the neuroprotective effects. In agreement with other laboratories, amyloid-beta peptides induced a rapid activation of c-Jun N-terminal kinase (JNK) by phosphorylation. Pre-treatment with aqueous LB extract markedly reduced the phosphorylation of JNK-1 (Thr183/Tyr185) and its substrates c-Jun-I (Ser 73) and c-Jun-II (Ser 63). Taken together, the results show potential neuroprotective effects of the extract from L. barbarum. Further studies on anti-aging herbal medicines like L. barbarum may open a new therapeutic window for the prevention of AD.

Synopsis. This study used in vitro techniques to determine whether wolfberry extracts could interfere with neurodegenerative effects of beta-amyloid, the protein commonly found post-mortem in the brains of Alzhemier's patients and thought to be a pathogen in Alzheimer's disease. Wolfberry extract did reduce metabolic stress by amyloid on isolated cortical neurons, indicating it may have protective effects under these controlled laboratory conditions. The study is very preliminary, however, showing that wolfberry constituents were counter-active to amyloid stress. As these experiments were conducted in vitro, it is inappropriate to conclude a definitive effect of wolfberry phytochemicals on amyloid's role in the living human with Alzheimer's disease.

Chapter Summary: Richness of Wolfberry Nutrients

We've seen in Chapters 3-6 the variety and concentrations of wolfberry phytonutrients with benefits these chemicals may impart to consumers of wolfberries. Although much of the research and conclusions about wolfberry health benefits are limited and premature, there is a collective favorable impression about the nutrient density in this berry to allow inference about health benefits to be gained by eating wolfberries.

What impresses most about wolfberries is the richness of nutrients packed into this plant. In Chapter 3, we presented the nutrients below which must be an incomplete list as research on wolfberries has not been extensive

- 18 amino acids
- 5 unsaturated ("heart healthy") fatty acids and at least one phytosterol
- 11 essential minerals
- 22 trace minerals
- vitamins A (via beta-carotene), C and E, and at least 3 B vitamins
- 6 monosaccharides and 8 polysaccharides
- 4 carotenoids
- and presence of antioxidant phenolic flavonoids, p-coumaric acid and scopoletin.

As a specific example of compounding nutrients to benefit a health function—a type of multinutrient synergy gained by eating whole berries rather than wolfberry extracts or juice—one can see that wolfberry's antioxidant vitamins, minerals, carotenoids, phenolics and polysaccharides fulfill such criteria.

Multiple antioxidant phytochemicals make wolfberry extraordinary among plants as perhaps the world's richest antioxidant food. This is a noteworthy compliment by itself.

But wolfberry provides such diverse nutrients in rich content that it deserves further investigation as perhaps Nature's single most nutritious food. At this point in our review, it seems reasonable to state that a more powerful nutritional source in Nature has not been described in the same detail as covered for wolfberries in this book.

Discussed in this Chapter were other newly-discovered wolfberry nutrients that are potentially beneficial, but with less understanding, including

- silybin-like pyrroles
- phenolic amides
- monomenthyl succinate
- scopoletin
- beta-sitosterol (daucosterol)
- p-coumaric acid
- ellagic acid
- betaine
- calystegines
- taurine
- terpenes which include beta-carotene—one of wolfberry's signature nutrients.

Further research is needed to fully define these interesting phytochemicals, their roles imparting health and other nutritional constituents yet to be identified in this bountiful plant.

Summary of Wolfberry Health Benefits from Juice Products

We have now reached a point of review on wolfberry science where we can comment on the claimed benefits of wolfberry juices, NingXia Red (a puree-enriched version of Berry Young Juice) and Goji Juice as mentioned in Chapter 2. Our aim is not to critique these popular products and their claims but rather objectively state evidence about wolfberry nutrients and potential health benefits from consuming the juice.

We hope to achieve this balance by reciting the proposed marketing claims then provide relevant scientific background to comment about the relationship. Further discussions about juice research and nutritional factors are presented in Chapter 10.

From Chapter 2, wolfberry juice (Goji Juice or NingXia Red Juice):

1. *Extends life, protects against premature aging, has powerful antioxidant actions*

In clinical science, a verified health benefit from a drug or food would have to be proven by the rigors of a clinical trial, as outlined in Chapter 2, to be accepted by scientific experts. The related effects of antioxidant protection against aging and gaining extended life that wolfberry consumption may offer are difficult to prove. It is probably safe to say that no such clinical research has actually been done to test these effects, but rather assumptions for prolonging youth and healthy life by eating wolfberries are based on Chinese myths and reputation.

The antioxidant benefits of wolfberries, however, are readily acceptable based on the science we now have, as richness in antioxidant phytochemicals is a signature characteristic of wolfberries (Chapter 5).

The above abstracts 13-15 of this chapter (others provided in the reference summary of Chapter 12) point to wolfberries affording improvements of memory (in mice), inhibition of apoptosis and increased synthesis or activity of antioxidant enzymes such as superoxide dismutase. Such effects combined with the compelling antioxidant values of carotenoids (Chapter 5) establish significant antioxidant qualities in wolfberries, but do not lead to conclusions about anti-aging or life-prolonging benefits in humans.

2. *Increases energy and strength*

As we saw in Chapter 3, wolfberries are an excellent source of carbohydrates and good fats providing significant caloric energy from a single serving. Monosaccharides and polysaccharides are important contributors to the carbohydrate content of wolfberries. There appear to be no studies specifically evaluating strength benefits from wolfberry consumption.

3. *Stimulates secretion of human growth hormone and promotes youthful appearance*

From the science reviewed, we were unable to verify an effect of wolfberries on growth hormone secretion or any systematic cosmetic benefits.

4. *Maintains healthy blood pressure*

In abstract 12, we saw that wolfberry polysaccharides appear significant for stimulating relaxation of vascular smooth muscle, possibly via formation of nitric oxide, the endothelium-derived relaxing factor (EDRF). In Chapter 3, we speculated that wolfberry's relatively high content of the amino acid, arginine, could be an important substrate for making nitric oxide and so contributing to blood pressure control. High potassium content from wolfberries is another potentially important contributor to regulation of blood pressure. However, there is no collective evidence from human studies to support this claim.

5. *Reduces blood cholesterol levels*

In Chapter 4, our hypothesis that wolfberry polysaccharides are metabolized in the intestinal system as fermentable fiber leads to a possibility that consuming wolfberries or wolfberry juice can reduce blood cholesterol levels. The main mechanisms of action would result from synthesis during fermentation of short-chain fatty acids that inhibit cholesterol synthesis in the liver and stimulate uptake of cholesterol from the blood. However, there is no collective evidence to support this evidence in people consuming wolfberries or its juice.

6. *Promotes normal blood sugar levels in diabetes mellitus*

Related to the effects explained above for cholesterol, formation of fatty acids from wolfberry polysaccharides as fermentable fiber would provide control of the glycemic response to a meal (reviewed in Chapter 4). Thus, there is good evidence for wolfberries contributing to regulation of blood glucose in diabetes, but human studies demonstrating this effect do not exist.

7. *Helps lose weight*

In a modest way, wolfberry consumption may contribute to weight control or loss. As a source of fermentable resistant starch (soluble dietary fiber) aiding to stabilize glucose levels and reduce appetite, wolfberry polysaccharides may indeed be important for this role. Dietary fiber, however, is not a singular macronutrient in the diet so does not act alone in determining body weight. Overall macronutrient volume and composition from other foods would be important for weight control. We found no systematic research addressing this topic so must conclude that such a benefit from wolfberry consumption is one of the myths.

8. *Enhances sexual functions and improves fertility*

Although this claim is one often stated with a long history in Chinese fables, it remains without any scientific foundation. There is no peer-reviewed published research to validate this claim.

9. *Relieves headaches and dizziness*

Another long-term reputed benefit from wolfberry's legend, there appears, however, to be no published research in which this effect was objectively studied.

10. *Relieves insomnia*

There is no peer-reviewed published research to validate this claim.

11. *Supports eye health*

Although no human study to date has specifically examined this claim for wolfberries, there is strong scientific evidence from nutrient isolation that eating wolfberries would benefit eye health. This effect is due mainly to the high comprehensive content of antioxidant nutrients in wolfberries—vitamins C and E (from leaves); minerals zinc, copper, selenium, manganese and magnesium; and antioxidant carotenoids and phenolics (Chapters 3,5). Particularly, the carotenoids zeaxanthin and lutein are absorbed selectively into the retina where they act as pigment filters and direct antioxidants (Chapter 5). Wolfberry's content of zeaxanthin per unit weight may be the highest among plants in Nature.

Although we emphasize that wolfberries naturally contain the AREDS nutrients (publications 25-29, Chapter 5) in amounts high for plants, the contents in wolfberries are not nearly adequate on a per serving basis to meet the supplement levels recommended for protection against age-related macular degeneration.

12. *Strengthens the heart and cardiovascular system*

Inferred by abstract 12 of this Chapter, wolfberry nutrients are likely a good foundation for health of the heart and cardiovascular system. Polysaccharides may have beneficial effects themselves but the more conventional heart-healthy nutrients—antioxidant compounds mentioned above—plus the omega-6 and -3 fatty acids and several essential minerals indicate that wolfberries have a complement of excellent constituents for maintaining cardiovascular health. To date, however, there is no collective evidence from human studies to support this claim..

13. *Improves disease resistance, strengthens immune responses, protects cellular DNA*

This category is probably the most intensively investigated area in wolfberry research, mainly due to the proposed immune enhancing properties of the polysaccharides (Chapter 4). The above statement goes too far, however, as there has been no clinical study demonstrating "disease resistance". Protection of DNA is assumed from preliminary in vitro studies, not conclusively proven. Nonetheless, several studies focused on various aspects of immune stimulation, collectively give strong indication that wolfberry polysaccharides (and probably other nutrients) contribute to immune health.

14. *Builds strong blood*

There is no peer-reviewed published research to validate this claim.

15. *Supports a healthy liver and pancreas*

Results from several experiments have been reported in which liver and pancreatic cells were used in vitro as model systems to test for activity of other biomarkers, such as enzyme activity. In clinical studies on humans, specific tests for normal liver and pancreas functions exist but these have not been applied to study organ-specific benefits of eating wolfberries. Consequently, it is not appropriate to extrapolate the benefits of wolfberries shown in bench top laboratory or animal tests to health or disease of the liver or pancreas in humans.

16. *Treats menopausal symptoms*

There is no peer-reviewed published research to validate this claim.

17. *Prevents morning sickness during the early phase of pregnancy*

There is no peer-reviewed published research to validate this claim.

18. *Strengthens muscles and bones*

There is no peer-reviewed published research to validate this claim.

19. *Improves memory*

In research summarized in Chapter 5, cognitive and anti-aging benefits are assumed but unproven by peer-reviewed published science. Consequently, this claim cannot be made as a benefit of wolfberry consumption.

20. *Supports normal kidney function*

There is no peer-reviewed published research to validate this claim.

21. *Relieves chronic cough*

There is no peer-reviewed published research to validate this claim.

22. *Alleviates anxiety and stress*

There is no peer-reviewed published research to validate this claim.

23. *Promotes cheerfulness*

There is no peer-reviewed published research to validate this claim.

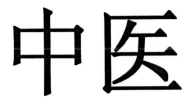

CHAPTER 7
Wolfberries And Traditional Chinese Medicine (TCM)

The first mention of wolfberries in Chinese legend is from a 2,000 year old book on its use as an herbal remedy for nourishing the yin and strengthening "qi" (pronounced "chee"), the body's energy well. It stated that wolfberry "replenishes the supply of body fluids, calms the spirit, refreshes the skin, brightens the complexion and strengthens the eyes."

The undocumented legend about wolfberries entering the diet for herbal remedies, however, is considerably older. It is thought to have existed at least since the time of Shen Nung, the first great Chinese herbalist who lived around 2,800 BC.

From the ancient Chinese myths, wolfberries have been used to treat impotence, dizziness, general weakness, fever, diabetes and numerous other health disorders. Other characteristics and applications mentioned in ancient texts:

- The root bark is considered bitter, cooling and antibacterial; bark has been used to control coughs and lower blood pressure and cholesterol, and to treat impotence, backache, sore throat, rheumatism and pneumonia.
- The dried berries and leaves have been used as a tea tonic to lower blood pressure and cholesterol; regular wolfberry tea consumption is thought to maintain healthy liver and kidney functions.
- Dried berry consumption has been used for controlling high blood pressure, weak eyes, vertigo, lumbago, impotence,

menopausal problems, chronic fevers, internal hemorrhage, nosebleed, tuberculosis, asthma and fatigue
- Its seed oils are popular for control of skin dryness, itching and as an antibiotic

Gaining a perspective on wolfberry's use in diets and TCM requires background to outline why plants are so revered in China to treat diseases and promote healthy life. In this chapter, we'll briefly review ancient Chinese cultural and dietary practices and early history of TCM, maintaining a focus on how eating a nutrient-rich food like wolfberries may impart health benefits.

Chinese Culture and the Five Elements

Like the well-known concept of yin and yang, the Five Elements Theory is a cornerstone of Chinese culture. Chinese followers of this theory believe people are surrounded by 5 energy fields—wood, fire, earth, metal, and water—that are not static but constantly moving, changing and interacting with one another.

Once theorists identified the five elements, they set about categorizing phenomena within the five categories. Everything, from a gentle waterfall to sounds of organs in our bodies, can be described in terms of the Five Elements. How things are characterized depends on individual qualities. For example, earth is associated with growth and nourishment, so the spleen, which stores and monitors blood—digesting red blood cell debris and producing white blood cells when necessary—is categorized as an earth element.

Just as an imbalance between yin and yang can produce unproductive forces, keeping the Five Elements in balance promotes harmony both in one's surroundings and among people. According to Chinese beliefs, each element acts upon at least two others, either stimulating it or controlling it. For example, wood evolves fire and controls or suppresses earth. Similarly, fire gives birth to earth and controls metal. All the elements are constantly interacting with other elements—none stands alone.

This background provides us with a foundation for understanding roles for wolfberries and choices among other foods for the diet.

The Five Elements in Feng Shui and Diet

The Five Elements theory enters many facets of Chinese life. In martial arts, for example, are several basic movements, each designed to keep the body in harmony with one of the elements and to control opposing forces. In Feng Shui, a current western trend in landscaping and interior decorating, the Five Elements are fundamentals. Literally meaning "wind and water," Feng Shui is concerned with alignment of energies in a home or work environment to have peaceful balance of surroundings and optimize personal energy.

For dietary practices, Chinese herbalists believe that a user needs to know the status of the Five Elements in her body. A deficiency or an excess of one element can lead to illness. In *The Chinese Kitchen: Recipes, Techniques, Ingredients, History, and Memories from America's Leading Authority on Chinese Cooking* (References), author Eileen Yin Fei-Lo provides numerous fascinating examples of how her grandmother used the principles of the Five Elements theory to prevent or treat common illnesses, while always making the diet interesting, colorful and nourishing as a basis for maintaining health. She mentions wolfberries and the plant's leaves and twigs as particularly good for making soups.

A detailed look at the use of Five Elements theory in diagnosing and treating illnesses is beyond our goals for this book. Let it be sufficient to say that practitioners of TCM rely on it to explain relationships between the body organs, diet, health and the outside environment.

Feng Shui Food Preparation

Ancient Chinese recipes show that balance in food can be achieved through use of colors. A plate full of food with bland or like colors presents a visually unappealing meal. By contrast, a stir-fry made with red wolfberries, yellow, green, red and orange bell peppers, purple eggplant, red tomatoes and lean meat would be a typical Feng Shui choice.

The concept of yin and yang also applies to food preparation, tastes and colors. Yin would provide milder flavors with subtle colors— wolfberries would likely be yin—while Yang would give bolder tastes and colors. Ancient Chinese recipes take advantage of this type of Feng Shui balance: sweet-sour, hot-sour, and strong flavored spicy dishes paired with plain rice are examples of yin/yang balanced foods. As wolfberries are red with a subtle, nutty taste, they readily find a place in Feng Shui food preparation.

Traditional Chinese Medicine (TCM)

TCM is an alternative or integrative system of medical treatment arising from a holistic philosophy of life. It emphasizes the interconnection of mental, emotional, and physical components within each person, and the importance of harmony between individuals and their social groups, as well as between humans and nature. Food is an important part of TCM, as one's choices for the diet are seen by practitioners as a way of preventing health problems.

In TCM, the practitioner seeks a solution dealing with the whole patient whereas the modern Western physician is often organ—or disease specific. Training of TCM physicians, therefore, involves all branches of the traditional "tree of therapy", including foods eaten. Simply, there exists no boundary between food and medicine in TCM, and wherever possible, the remedy for health problems is sought first through nutrition.

We emphasize this here as a way of drawing the reader back to the purpose of the book and contents of Chapters 2-6. That is, wolfberry is such a nutritious food that its use in TCM must have been a natural selection over the ages to probe for possible health effects. It certainly seems justified now that its nutrient content is better understood.

Also part of TCM practice is to emphasize consumption of raw foods, sometimes several together, to prevent diseases or treat diagnosed problems. Later in Chapter 10, we detail various factors in fruit processing that affect phytochemical density and quality, and so indirectly support the intuitive belief that raw foods are preferred to gain optimal nutrient content.

TCM is not the only form of herbal therapy practiced today, nor is it the oldest—the ancient Indian medicine called Ayurvedic seems to hold that distinction. TCM is, however, the oldest *continuous tradition of herbal medicine* and is the basis for alternative and integrative medicine in many parts of the World.

In 1970 the Chinese Academy of Medical Science published a collection of traditional herbal remedies in common use. It lists some 800 prescriptions made from over 200 plant or animal ingredients. A group of American pharmacologists evaluated these prescriptions by modern biochemical analysis in 1974 and estimated that 45% are valid and useful.

TCM Purpose

The purpose of TCM is to restore health through correction of imbalances within the patient's body or between the patient and the larger social and natural order. TCM regards the human body as a small-scale reflection of the Universe, with principles of treatment derived from Taoism, the ancient Chinese philosophy emphasizing one to follow the right path (the "Tao) in order to find harmony within the Universe.

Taoism's holistic emphasis was reflected in the close correlation between TCM and daily dietary habits. In Chinese herbal legend, foods were eaten for their therapeutic qualities and adjusted to changes in the body to cure illnesses or maintain day-to-day health over a lifetime.

The specific teachings of Taoism that have had the most profound effect on Chinese medicine are the concept of duality and belief in the primordial form of universal energy, *qi*. The terms yin and yang are applied to the two primal opposites that continually interact and produce constant change in the Universe and one's body, and so are intimately linked to diet.

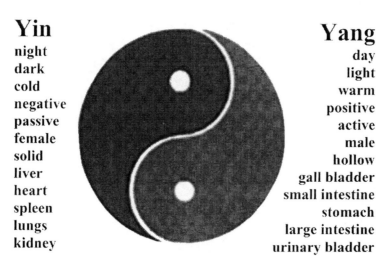

Yin	Yang
night	day
dark	light
cold	warm
negative	positive
passive	active
female	male
solid	hollow
liver	gall bladder
heart	small intestine
spleen	stomach
lungs	large intestine
kidney	urinary bladder

Yin Yang, an underlying principle of Chinese philosophy and medicine. Good health is believed to come from a balance of Yin (negative, dark, and feminine) and Yang (positive, bright, and masculine). From the History of Medicine Division, US National Library of Medicine, Bethesda, MD

Yang is associated with heat, dryness, brightness, upward or outward movement, forceful action, lightness, and speed. Yin represents the corresponding qualities of cold, moisture, dimness, downward or inward movement, quietness, heaviness, and slowness. These opposites are regarded as interdependent rather than mutually destructive or antagonistic. Humans participate in *qi*—the universal life force which Taoism believes circulates throughout the body and determines a person's basic level of vitality.

Over centuries, Chinese TCM doctors worked out elaborate systems of correlation between 1) yin and yang and the Five Elements (wood, fire, earth, metal, and water); 2) ten major internal organs of the body; and 3) meridians, or invisible three-dimensional pathways that circulate *qi* and blood throughout the body. Taoism believes the meridians regulate the body's yin/yang balance, providing connections between the person and cosmic forces, and protecting the body against external sources of disease. Prescriptions for herbal medicines are formulated to correct excesses of yin or yang, incorrect flow of *qi*, disorders located in a specific organ, or emotional problems that accompany physical illness. According to TCM, these factors are extensions of what one consumes as food.

There seems to be no boundary between food and body functions in TCM, and wherever possible, food is used as a preventive practice.

Written around 650 AD by the Tang dynasty physician, Sun Sze Miao, "The physician first treats the patient with food; only when food fails does he resort to medicines." He also said "An experienced doctor anticipates and treats patients for the unseen diseases" (meaning before they reveal as symptoms), whereas "the inexperienced doctor treats patients for their seen diseases".

Synopsis of TCM Practice

Diagnosis

Diagnosis in TCM has four phases:
- Visual examination. The doctor notes the patient's expression, complexion, and general physique. The distinctive feature of Chinese medicine is the detailed examination of the tongue for color, shape, and coating (if any).
- Listening/smelling. The TCM doctor listens to the breathing and looks for any unusual body sounds or odors.
- Verbal questions. This phase is similar to history-taking in a western medical examination. Focus is placed on what the patient has been eating.
- Palpation. The TCM doctor feels the patient's organs through

the abdomen, the *qi* points along the meridians, and the pulse. Pulse diagnosis is given special attention in the Chinese system and is regarded by patients as an important measure of a doctor's skill.

TCM Treatment

TCM is highly individualized because the practitioner proceeds from the assumption that different individuals have different *qi* and therefore various degrees of vulnerability to internal imbalances or external causes of disease. TCM generally offers the patient several ways to receive therapy and rebalance *qi,* including use of herbs and nutrition, exercise and meditation, acupuncture and massage. All these methods are viewed in TCM as synergistic and harmonious with one another.

External treatments. TCM applies herbs to the body externally as well as internally. Dried herbs may be mixed with water and used as poultices to treat arthritis, rheumatism, sprains, bruises, abscesses, and strained backs. Acupuncture, massage, and the use of suction cups are external treatments often used in TCM in conjunction with internal herbal therapy.

Internal treatments. TCM uses herbs for preventive treatment as well as for curing illness. Prescriptions are fine-tuned by an herbalist, as well as by the TCM doctor, and formulated according to the patient's condition, as well as the nature of the herbs. When a patient takes the doctor's prescription to the herbalist, it will be made up in one of several traditional forms: broth, pills, wine with herbs steeped in it, gum, fermented dough, or paste. Pills may be made with wax, honey, or flour pastes that may be used externally or internally.

This is where wolfberries most likely had their origin as internal treatments in TCM.

Early Founders of Herbal Medicine

The development of TCM follows the *written* course of Chinese civilization, a history of some 5,000 years.

The first herbal medicines can be traced to Emperor Shen Nung (pronounced "shay-noon"), the "Divine Husbandman," who lived circa 2800 BC. As father of Chinese agriculture, he is one of three legendary providers for the Chinese nation; the others are Fu Xi, the first animal farmer, and Shui Ren, founder of fire.

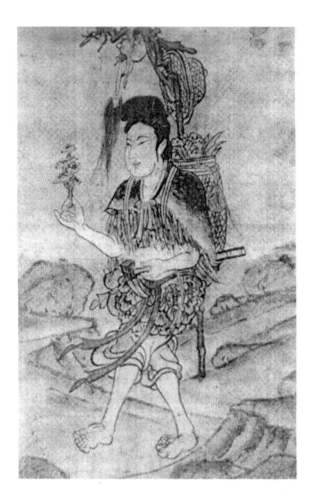

Shen Nung, circa 2800 BC, from Studies on Lycium barbarum, China Scientific Book Services, 1999.

An explorer and perhaps the first to record plant taxonomy, Shen Nung experimented on hundreds of herbs to understand their nutritive and healing effects. Legend has it that he made drawings, descriptions and concoctions of several hundred plants, minerals and animal extracts, many of which he tested on himself.

A berry with wolfberry's characteristics is mentioned in records attributed to Shen Nung.

The plants described were divided into three categories—superior, medium, and inferior—determined by their rejuvenating, tonic, or curative properties. Since the rejuvenating plants were deemed superior, prevention seemed more highly regarded than curing in this ancient form of TCM practiced by Shen Nung, a simple strategy of TCM practiced today.

His records were handed down by story-telling from generation to generation over 29 centuries. They were interpreted in part from drawings and symbols found on ox bones and turtle shells used as "books" of the time and excavated in the 20th century.

Eventually, these records were interpreted as the medical diaries ("materia medica") of the Divine Husbandman—Shen Nung, *Pen Ts'ao Ching*—*Materia Medica of the Divine Husbandman*. They must have been handed down through fables for about 3,000 years and were finally written into the book, author unknown, around 200 AD, Han Dynasty.

The first volume of this work includes drawings of herbs, minerals, and animals. The remaining volumes cover the pharmaceutical and therapeutic uses of the materia medica, and remain an historical treasure of perhaps the origin of TCM.

Shen Nung's portrait and records are on display at Johns Hopkins University Hospital in Baltimore. A website describing him and other Chinese legends, including portrait drawings, is maintained by the US National Library of Medicine, National Institutes of Health (see chapter references). Venerated as a Father of TCM, Shen Nung is also believed to have first used tea leaves for making a recreational beverage and introducing the technique of acupuncture.

Shen Nung's discovery of tea drinking provides a glimpse for how this practice of taste-testing plants began.

Once after a long forest walk examining plants randomly, Shen Nung was about to drink some water he had boiled, when a few leaves from an overhanging tree blew into the pan. Deciding to taste this unlikely brew, Shen Nung discovered what tea-drinkers the world over know today—tea from leaves was delicious, refreshing and provided a calming effect possibly linked to bioactive herbs.

It is likely wolfberries or its leaves were also used as an herb source for early teas; wolfberry fruit and leaves for tea are perhaps the most popular beverage application of the plant by country peasants in China.

The well-known *Yellow Emperor's Classic of Medicine* (*Hung Di Nei Jing*) is the work of the Warring States Period from 475 BC to 221 BC. Bian Chueh compiled the *Difficult Classic* (*Nan Jing*) to supplement the

Hung Di Nei Jing. Another major work of this period is the *Classic of Mountain and Sea*, which described 270 plants, animals and minerals with medicinal effects.

TCM made a significant leap forward during the Han Dynasty (200 BC to 220 AD)—one of the most prosperous periods in China's early history. *Shen Nung's Materia Medica* was compiled late in this period. Zhang Zong Jing (150-219 A.D.) wrote two highly revered books still used as ancient references today: *Summaries of Common Diseases* (*Jing Kuei Yao Lueh*) and *Discussion of Cold-Induced Disorders* (*Shang Han Lun*).

TCM reached another height in the Tang Dynasty (618 to 907 AD). The royal government established the Imperial Medical College in 624 AD to oversee further research and teaching of TCM, more than 200 years before the first medical college was established anywhere in the Western world.

Sun Sze Miao (590-682 AD) was one of the most accomplished scholars in this period. He wrote *Thousand Precious Formulas* and *Thousand Precious Supplemental Formulas*, detailing herbal prescriptions and acupuncture meridians.

In 659 AD the Tang government commissioned Su Jing and his colleagues to revise the *New Materia Medica*, the first official pharmacopoeia in the world.

Blossom of a Thousand Flowers

The progress of TCM during the Sung (962-1279), Yuan (1215-1368), Ming (1368-1644) and Ching (1644-1911) Dynasties was unprecedented—a thousand year period sometimes called the "Blossom of a Thousand Flowers" when typesetting played a major role in recording and publishing information, allowing numerous schools of thoughts to be recorded, published, disseminated and debated, including many documents of TCM.

The first Imperial Pharmacy was founded by the Sung Court in 1151. Chen Shi Wen and his colleagues compiled *Formulas of Imperial People's Pharmacy*, a revision of *Tai Ping Royal Formulas* that lists over 20,000 formulas in 1,700 categories, many of which were established on herbal remedies.

The most celebrated herbal work is Li Shi Zhen's (1518-1593) *Grand Materia Medica* published after his death during the Ming Dynasty in 1596. It has 52 volumes describing 1,892 plants and extracts and 8,160 formulas. Li Shi Zhen is regarded as China's greatest herbalist, but clearly his work extended from the foundation established by Shen Nung 4,300 years earlier.

TCM went through a period of decline in the late 18th century during the Russian invasion of China. The occupation worsened conditions for China during the 19th century, with Japan also invading from the northeast and Western imperialists from the south. A series of military and political defeats, including the First Opium War (1839-1842), the Anglo-Franco Invasion (1856-1860) and Boxer Rebellion (1900-1901) brought China into deeper despair. Losing vast territories, priceless national treasures, and confidence in many of its old values, China became skeptical of the "unscientific" TCM in the early 1900s and its practices were mostly discontinued.

TCM was attacked by pro-Western reformists and supporters of Western-style medicine. The attack climaxed in 1928 when the Nationalist Government proposed to end TCM licensing. As a protest, however, on March 17, 1929, some 300 TCM delegates presented an appeal to Chiang Kai Shek, chairman of the Military Committee and Chinese National Minister of Public Health. Kai Shek eventually overturned legislation against TCM, this date ending the dark period of TCM history and becoming a national holiday still continued for celebrating TCM..

Renaissance and Influence of Dr. Cui Yueli, 1930-2000

In 1931, a wealthy American traveler named G.M. Gest was cured from an eye disease by a Chinese TCM physician after all other efforts had failed. Over following years, Gest, motivated by gratitude and a new appreciation of TCM, collected thousands of books (eventually 75,000!) about Chinese medicine and established the Gest Oriental Library at Princeton University in New Jersey. It exists today as probably the world's greatest collection of TCM history and practices.

In 1977, *Zhong Yao Da Ci Dian* (Encyclopedia of Chinese Materia Medica) was published by the Jiangsu Institute of New Medicine. It is the most comprehensive Chinese TCM materia medica in the world, consisting of three volumes with a total of 3,588 pages. The book describes 5,767 herbal drugs with 4,500 drawings, many in great detail. This book also includes chemical structures of compounds or isolates of drugs described in the encyclopedia.

Over the 1970s and 80s, the Chinese Ministry of Health was under leadership of several TCM advocates, notably Dr. Cui Yueli who systematically created new TCM colleges across China. Western medical science courses were added to the curriculum, establishing foundation for a new field later called *integrative medicine*. Graduates received advanced science and medical degrees to recognize their academic and social status.

A significant development at this time was the insertion of TCM teaching into major medical universities in China. This marriage between Eastern and Western medicine gave further support for integrative medicine acknowledging TCM as an effective adjunct to modern medical science.

Credit for the overall renaissance of TCM is given to China's Chairman at this time, Mao Tse Tung who proclaimed "Traditional Chinese Medicine is a great national treasure. It must be thoroughly studied and elevated to a higher level."

When political and economic relations between China and the US eased, TCM was reintroduced to the US and other Western countries. Its popularity increased substantially over following decades, as a number of TCM colleges formed across the US and Canada where the number of TCM practitioners increased more than tenfold by 2000. China has played an important role by providing its own TCM scholars and clinicians to become the backbone of TCM education and practices worldwide.

In the US since the mid-1990s, the National Institutes of Health established the **National Center for Complementary and Alternative Medicine** with an annual budget of more than $250 million. Some major medical schools in the US have created offices for integrative medicine, having a mission to perpetuate blending Eastern and Western medical practices, first started in China more than 50 years ago.

Cui Yueli Research Center for TCM

Cui Yueli Research Center (CYRC) for TCM, Beijing (picture), was named after Dr. Cui Yueli, Vice or First Minister of Health for China from 1978-87, and an influential government leader for the TCM renaissance. Dr. Cui was a highly respected physician and traditional herbalist who dedicated himself to perpetuating TCM.

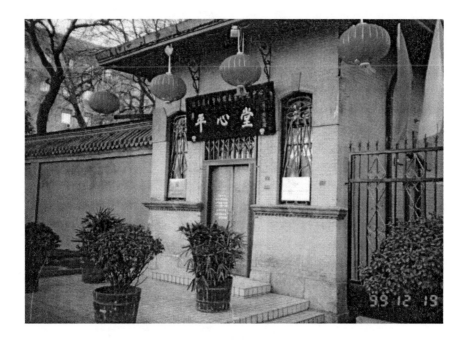

At CYRC, there is an herbal remedy collection of 50 TCM masters plus a network of over 700 TCM practitioners nationwide registered with the State Bureau of TCM. The mission of CYRC is to discover the treasure of experience and practice of TCM over the centuries, and to combine it with modern science. There are hundreds of the most effective herbal formulas defined at the center, with many of these under current research to validate them scientifically.

Wolfberry is a popular main ingredient in many of these formulas to treat heart disease, the immune system, sexual dysfunction, fatigue, vertigo, tinnitus, visual degeneration, headaches, insomnia, chronic liver diseases, diabetes, and a variety of other possible health applications implied from its use over history. Some of these references were presented in Chapters 4-6. Wolfberries remain under active research at CYRC.

The Cui Yueli TCM Research Center is a privately owned clinic and research facility established in 1998 for the memory of Dr. Cui Yueli who died that year. Dr. Cui dedicated his life to the heritage and development of TCM, and aimed to spread it globally.

During his term as Minister of Health, he raised financial interests to promote the Chinese TCM network, expanding the number of traditional clinics from 100 to more than 1000. He traveled extensively across China to visit villages and shamans with intent to record, preserve and develop their traditional practices, encouraging that authentic procedures be passed on to younger TCM practitioners.

Dr. Cui supported scientific research on TCM hypotheses and urged integration with western medicine. His ultimate wish was to validate and further develop TCM into common practice within the new field of integrative medicine, placing China in a position for TCM leadership around the World.

The Clinic of the Center has trained TCM doctors providing acupuncture, traditional herbal therapies and Tuina (Chinese massage) treatment for patients. CYRC continues today with a broad range of herbal research projects involving academic centers in Beijing.

TCM is embraced by the general population of China. Despite the widespread growth of western medicine in China over the past century, medicine in the Chinese countryside is still dominated by TCM, particularly in treating chronic and rare diseases.

Compilation of a *Chinese Medicine Classic Series*, a TCM compendium expected for completion this decade, is one of the main tasks of CYRC. This series written in modern simplified Chinese will contain over 30 million characters to be translated into English and other languages. The series consists of the original classics in TCM used for training new TCM physicians.

Dr. Cui planned and organized this project himself in 1997. His untimely death in 1998 left the project unfinished, but the task has been adopted by many in China determined to see TCM flourish as Cui Yueli had wished.

Biography of Cui Yueli, 1920-1998 (also see Dedication)

- 1938-1949: military officer and medical training
- 1964-1966: Deputy Mayor, Beijing
- 1978-1982: Federal Vice Minister of Health
- 1981-1987: Director, Chinese Society of Combined Traditional and Western Medicine
- 1981-1998: Chairman, Traditional Chinese Medical Association, China
- 1982-1987: Federal Minister of Health
- 1985: National Chairman, Red Cross Society

植物

CHAPTER 8
Botanical Taxonomy For Wolfberry,
Lycium Barbarum L.

Our goal in this chapter is to outline the taxa for wolfberry, giving enough specificity about its botanical origin and growing characteristics to allow an understanding of its plant relatives. Through this background, we hope to give the reader a perspective on factors that make wolfberry such an extraordinary nutritional source.

Wolfberry is known by several synonym names: Fructus lycii (Lycium fruit), goji or gouji fruit, ningxia gou qi, gou qi zi (fruit), di gu pi (bark), gou qi ye (leaves), Lycium chinense (Miller), kukoshi (Japanese), kugicha (Korean), kau kei chi (Cantonese), matrimony vine, Duke of Argyll's tea plant, Chinese boxthorn, morali, murali, Christmas berry.

Among native Chinese and Chinese-Americans, gou qi zi ("goji") from Ningxia is the most highly prized wolfberry fruit. A common synonym hybrid of Lycium barbarum L. in Ningxia is Lycium halimifolium (Miller).

Wolfberry's scientific or formal botanical name, *Lycium barbarum L.*, has historical and Latin derivatives:

- *Lycium*—possibly from the ancient nation of "Lydia", a former country of Asia Minor first mentioned by Homer in the 8th century BC or from the Latin, lychnus, meaning "light" or "lamp", perhaps due to the oval shape of the wolfberry fruit
- *barbarum*—Latin for "foreign" (from the outside) or may refer to the ancient country of Barbary, formerly part of northern Africa

- *L.* derives from Carl Linnaeus, the Swedish botanist who established taxonomic nomenclature in the 1700s still in use today to specify plant species individually

Linnaeus is credited with devising the modern binomial system of plant scientific names using a genus first name and a specie second name, *Lycium barbarum,* used the first time for wolfberry apparently in 1753.

To know a plant's taxa is to know its immediate plant family and distant relatives, growing dispositions and habits, likes, dislikes, "friends", "enemies", etc.

Considering an example familiar to most readers, broccoli, cabbage, and Brussels sprouts all belong to the Cruciferae or mustard family. One can assume they have similar growing needs: full sun, plenty of water, soil acidity near neutral but high in fertility, and so on. All tolerate cold weather, dislike prolonged heat, prefer regular but light moisture and are susceptible to beetles and crucifer worms. We'll look at some of these characteristics for wolfberry in this chapter.

A plant's full pedigree starts with its membership in the plant kingdom. From there, taxonomists apply ever more rigorous classification names to specify a given plant's taxa—its specific classifications in the order of plants that define a specie as unique. We will detail the taxa below for wolfberry.

For further orientation, a close relative of the wolfberry in the Solanaceae family—the eggplant—has fruit that is actually a large berry with the same shape and growth stages as wolfberry's fruit. Its division within the plant kingdom is Spermatophyte (also for wolfberry), meaning that it doesn't produce by simple cell division but generates by seeds rather than spores. Further, eggplant is assigned (as is wolfberry) to the class Angiospermae, a flowering plant. Its Angiospermae subclass (like wolfberry) is Dicotyledonae, meaning that two leaves, rather than one, sprout from its seed.

Eggplant's and wolfberry's taxonomic order is Solanales, i.e., having both male and female organs in five-petaled flowers and sharing other characteristics, like alternate leaves and fragrant blossoms.

Most popular taxonomy guides zero in on the next levels down: suborder and family. The suborder for eggplant and wolfberry is Solanum, a broad grouping that includes ornamental plants like African holly and poisonous species of the common nightshades and Jerusalem cherries.

Solanum includes great variety of herbs, shrubs, trees, and vines, having 1400+ species in this suborder.

The genus for wolfberry is given next as the first word in the botanical binomial—*Lycium*, pertaining to deciduous and evergreen shrubs that are often spiny and grow in a variety of landscapes (this diversity is sometimes called "cosmopolitan") in temperate, maritime and even subtropical regions around the world.

After genus, the second word in the botanical binomial is the *specific epithet* defining a species, e.g., *Lycium barbarum*. This is what sets one plant apart from another within the same genus. A specific epithet may be a noun or an adjective. It may indicate a distinguishing characteristic of structure or flower color in the species.

Elatus, for example, is an adjective meaning tall. It may indicate something about the habitat where a species happens to flourish. *Palustris* is an adjective meaning "from swampy places" so common Palustris species prefer wet spongy habitats.

For wolfberry, *barbarum* was assigned to indicate its apparently "foreign" origin to where it was growing at the time of discovery.

That's the end of the botanist's job in name assignment but horticulturists add another category, called "varietal" or "cultivar" (cv), for cultivated variety, such as Lycium barbarum Chinese cv (Miller). A cultivar may be ascribed to a particular genus or, if of hybrid or unknown origin, just to a genus, similar to the many varietals of Lycium relatives in the USA as shown below under "Species".

Here we'll list in descending order the taxa of wolfberry as a specie of the Lycium genus:

1. **Kingdom: Plantae**—Plants
2. **Subkingdom: Tracheobionta**—Vascular plants
3. **Superdivision: Spermatophyta**—Plants with seeds
4. **Division: Magnoliophyta**—Plants that flower
5. **Class: Magnoliopsida**—Dicotyledons, or flowering plants with two embryonic seed leaves or "cotyledons" appearing at germination
6. **Subclass: Asteridae**—herbs, trees and shrubs having 2 fused carpels
7. **Order: Solanales or Solanum**—annuals, perennials, sub-shrubs, shrubs and climbers, often having attractive fruit and

flowers. Many are poisonous, but several bear edible fruit, such as the common foods tomato, potato, eggplant and wolfberry.

8. **Superfamily: Solanaceae**—"Potato family", nightshades with wide diversity such as paprika, chili pepper, tobacco, tomato, eggplant and petunia. They are shrubs, usually spiny, with deciduous or evergreen alternate, simple leaves 1-8 cm long. The flowers are solitary or in small clusters, 6-25 mm diameter, with a corolla of five purple, white or greenish-white petals joined together at their bases. The fruit is sometimes a red, purple or black berry 8-20 mm diameter (eggplant larger), similar to a nightshade or bittersweet berry.

9. **Genus: Lycium**—desert-thorn or boxthorn, a genus of about 100 species of plants native throughout many subtropical, desert and temperate zones of the world.

10. **Species: Lycium barbarum**—wolfberry

In the United States, there are 21 other varietals/cultivars of Lycium growing in nearly every state as listed by the US Department of Agriculture: L. andersonii (water jacket), L. berlandieri (Berlandieri's wolfberry), L. californicum (California desert-thorn), L. carolinianum (Carolina desert-thorn), L. chinense (Chinese desert-thorn), L. cooperi (peach thorn), L. exertum (Arizona desert-thorn), L. ferrocissimum (African boxthorn), L. fremontii (Fremont's desert-thorn), L. hassei (Santa Catalina Island desert-thorn), L. macrodon (desert wolfberry), L. pallidum (pale desert-thorn), L. parishii (Parish's desert-thorn), L. puberulum (downy desert-thorn), L. richii (Baja desert-thorn), L. sandwicense (Hawaii desert-thorn), L. shockleyi (Shockley's desert-thorn), L. texanum (Texas desert-thorn), L. torreyi (Torrey wolfberry), L. tweedianum (tropical desert-thorn), L. verrucosum (San Nicholas desert-thorn). In Canada, wolfberry is being cultivated on specialized farms in south-central British Columbia.

Lycium dasystemum (Pojark) and Lycium Chinese (Miller) var. potaninii (Pojark) are also considered major hybrids of Lycium barbarum in China.

Summary Characteristics of Wolfberry, Lycium barbarum L. (see wolfberry pictures on front and back covers)

General description—A perennial shrub with long, weak, thorny arched or climbing vines (picture) bearing short hairs, 1-6 m tall, often forming dense, tangled bushes in the wild. Shrub is exceptionally hardy with a long natural life possibly exceeding 100 years.

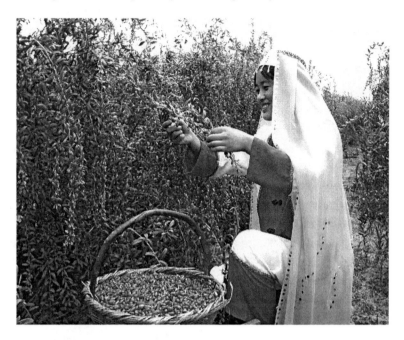

Leaves—Alternate or in bundles of up to 3 short-stalked entire, dull, elliptic to lanceolate (shaped like a lance, longer than it is wide) or ovate (egg-like in shape), up to 7 cm long and 3.5 cm wide on strong young shoots. The tips are blunted or round.

Flowers—About 1-3 from leaf axils on stalks 0.7 to 2 cm long. Calyx, bell-shaped to tubular, ruptured by the growing fruit, 3-6 lobes short and triangular. Corolla lavender or purplish, 9-14 cm long with 5-6 broad spreading lobes shorter than or equaling the tube. Anthers open length-wise, shorter than the filaments. Flowering time—June-Sept.

Fruits—Berries, fleshy, juicy, ellipsoid or oblong, 1-2 cm long, bright red (see front cover). Seeds, 20-30 per berry, compressed with curved embryo. Maturation Aug-Oct.

Germination—Dormancy in wolfberry seeds is variable. Seed samples of Anderson wolfberry and Arizona desert-thorn germinated well without pretreatment. They had germination success rates of 68% and 94%, respectively. Germination of matrimony vine seeds, however, was hastened and improved by stratification in moist sand for 60 to 120 days at 5 °C. After cold stratification, the average germination capacity for 19 samples was 74%. These tests were run in sand flats for 30 to 40 days at diurnally alternating temperatures of 30 to 20 °C. Germination after 18 days was 54%.

Soil preferences—Wolfberry prefers light sandy soils along riverbanks but is a hardy plant successful under a variety of growing conditions. It prefers a well-drained moist soil with alkaline (pH 8.0) to neutral (pH 7.4) acidity. It can grow in semi-shade, such as partial woodland, but is often successful in full sun exposure.

Habitat, ecosystem and climate—On river flood plains, low mountain slopes, wastelands, fields, roadsides, ditches, abandoned fields and homesteads, and as wall climbers near homes or farm buildings. Succeeds in maritime exposures.

Exposed to wide temperature ranges over the year in Ningxia from extreme winter cold- 20 °C to high summer heat +35 °C. Summers tend to be dry and sunny with total annual sunshine between 2200 and 3100 hours. Diurnal range of temperature from 12 °C to 15 °C, although 25 °C to 35 °C is common in summer.

Has considerable underlying cover by herbaceous species. Typically has standing biomass and litter accumulation and constituent shrub species also capable of continual reproduction by seed.

Collection of fruits; extraction and storage of seeds—Ripe berries may be picked from the vines in late summer to early fall. The berries are soft and juicy so usually require careful hand-picking. They may be pulped by forcing them through a screen and floating out the pulp.

For extraction and puree preparation on a larger scale, berries may be fermented, mashed in water, and then run through a mill equipped with screens of suitable sizes. Whole berries air-dried under gentle heat yield excellent raisin-like fruit for snacks and diverse uses in meals and beverages.

A method for seed isolation is to soak the berries until soft (usually over-night) then divide them from the fruit pulp with tweezers while holding the berry under water. Seeds that float are discarded as they are generally not viable. Remaining seeds are then dried and packaged air-tight until ready to plant. Usually one berry yields 20-30 viable seeds.

Seeds can be planted either in flats and transplanted later to pots or individually seeded into cells. Germination procedures are similar to methods used for tomatoes. Seedling emergence is generally 8-10 days depending on whether started in a greenhouse, coldframe, or stratified in moist sand.

Stratified wolfberry seeds will maintain good viability for 6 months, but there is no information on long-term storage of dry seeds. Methods for seed preservation appear to be orthodox, however, so storage should not be a problem.

Regeneration and successional status—Virtually all recovery in the wild is dependent upon seed germination and propagation by birds and nectar-seeking insects

Distribution—Native to Chinese regions of Ningxia, Anhui, Fujian, Gansu, Guangdong, Guangxi, Guizhou, Hainan, North Hebei, Heilongjiang, Henan, Hubei, Hunan, Jiangsu, Jiangxi, Jilin, Liaoning, Nei Mongol, Qinghai, North Shanxi, Sichuan, Tianjin Shi, Xinjiang, Yunnan and Zhejiang. Widely cultivated and naturalized in Europe, USA and throughout Asia (Japan, Korea, Nepal, Pakistan).

Conservation planning—Conversion to grassland accomplished by repeated burning in successive or alternate years.

Horticultural uses—As an informal hedge, succeeding in a wide variety of exposures, such as desert, subtropical, maritime. Has an extensive root system and can be planted to stabilize sandy river banks.

Natural enemies, pests, pathogens—aphids, red spiders and Paratrioza; see Table 10, Chapter 9 for other pests

Phytological Fingerprints—In their book on wolfberries (they say "goji" berries, Chapter 2 references), Mindell and Handel describe "fingerprints" of wolfberries from different Chinese growing regions as important characteristics for berry quality. The authors cite the Fourier Transform Infrared Spectral (FTIS) signature as an objective method for identifying these characteristics (see below references retrieved from PubMed).

Study Claim. A DNA analysis is used to differentiate the genetic fingerprint of one wolfberry specie from another.

1. **Publication.** Planta Med. 2001 Jun;67(4):379-81. **Differentiation of Lycium barbarum from its related Lycium species using random amplified polymorphic DNA.** Zhang KY, Leung HW, Yeung HW, Wong RN.

Abstract. The RAPD (random amplified polymorphic DNA) technique was applied for the first time to distinguish Lycium barbarum from other closely related species of the same genus. In this study, eight samples were collected, including five species, two varieties and one cultivated variety. A total of fifty arbitrary primers were used in the RAPD analysis. Distinctive DNA fingerprints corresponding to different Lycium species were successfully obtained from ten primers. Similarity index (S.I.) analysis revealed that the values are higher between intraspecies than interspecies. These results confirmed that the RAPD technique can be employed for distinguishing closely related species of Lycium.

Synopsis. Although this study indicates distinct genetic fingerprints exist between species of wolfberries, there is no identification of the molecular sources of these fingerprints. Whether the spectra represent polysaccharide differences, as Mindell and Handel suggest, or other phytochemicals in wolfberries, was not determined.

2. Publication. Guang Pu Xue Yu Guang Pu Fen Xi. 2003 Jun;23(3):509-11. **[FTIR and classification study on gouqi from different cultural areas]** [Article in Chinese] Zhou Q, Sun SQ, Leung HW. Department of Chemistry, Tsinghua University, Beijing, China.

Abstract. Gouqi (i.e., wolfberry), a commonly used traditional Chinese medicine, was studied by Fourier transform infrared (FTIR) spectroscopy. The combination of FTIR with mathematic method was used for the first time to classify the Gouqi from different cultivation areas. It can be seen that the Gouqi samples from Ningxia Yuxi, Ningxia Zhongning and Neimenggu Tuoketuoqi could be successfully classified by soft independent modeling of class analogy (SIMCA). As having fast and accurate characters, FTIR provides a new way to evaluate the origin of the Chinese medicines objectively based on the traditional methods.

Synopsis. This research is likely the same as that sourced by Mindell and Handel to discuss Fourier spectroscopy for differentiating wolfberries from different growing regions of China (Chapter 9).

3. Publication. Guang Pu Xue Yu Guang Pu Fen Xi. 2004 Jun;24(6):679-81. **[A rapid method for identification of genus lycium by FTIR spectroscopy]** [Article in Chinese] Peng Y, Sun SQ, Zhao ZZ, Leung HW. School of Chinese Medicine, Hong Kong Baptist University, Hong Kong, China.

Abstract. In this article, a newer method than above of using

Fourier-transform infrared spectroscopy (FTIR) to identify 7 species and 3 variations of genus lycium (Gouqi or wolfberry) in China is described. This method is based on the additive IR absorptions of the chemical components and the differences of their relative contents in various Gouqi. These differences are reflected in the FTIR spectra. The method provides a novel fingerprinting technique for the identification and differentiation of traditional Chinese medicine. Such technique can serve as a rapid, simple, reliable and non-destructive analytical method for Gouqi as a Chinese material medication.

Other current research, 2003-present:

4. **Publication.** Cell Biol Int. 2005 Jan;29(1):71-5. Epub 2005 Jan 26. **Transfer of transformed chloroplasts from Nicotiana tabacum to the Lycium barbarum plants.** Sytnik E, Komarnytsky I, Gleba Y, Kuchuk N. Institute of Cell Biology & Genetic Engineering, Kyiv, Ukraine.

Abstract. Plastid transformation is an attractive technology for obtaining crop plants with new useful characteristics and for fundamental researches of plastid functioning and nuclear-plastid interaction. The aim of our experiments was to obtain plants with Lycium barbarum nucleus and transformed Nicotiana tabacum plastids. Plastome of previously engineered transplastomic tobacco plants contains reporter uidA gene and selective aadA gene that confers resistance to antibiotics spectinomycin and streptomycin. Asymmetric somatic hybridization was performed for transferring transformed tobacco plastids from transplastomic tobacco plants into recipient L. barbarum wild type plants. Hybrid L. barbarum plants containing transformed tobacco plastome with active aadA and uidA genes were obtained as a result of the experiments. The work shows the possibility of obtaining transplastomic plants by transferring the transformed plastids to remote species by using somatic hybridization technology. The developed technique is especially effective for obtaining transplastomic plants that have low regeneration and transformation ability

Synopsis. This study examined the ability for transferring genetic characteristics from tobacco to wolfberries (related in the Solanaceae family), a method that may insert improved growing factors into recipient plants.

Although we present only these four current research interests on the family tree of wolfberry, there is certainly a great deal more under current investigation in China and elsewhere. As wolfberry's story becomes better known by the public and perhaps studied more intensively by plant and food scientists, its scientific foundations for horticulture and nutrition will strengthen in coming years.

耕作

CHAPTER 9
Wolfberry Cultivation, Harvesting and Geography

Wolfberries have grown in China since the beginning of recorded time several thousands of years ago, noted in the earliest herbal medical practices by the Divine Husbandman and father of Chinese horticulture, Shen Nung (circa 2800 BC).

Harvested now as an emerging economic opportunity for many Chinese food and beverage products, wolfberries are grown in several regions of China as well as other countries attracting export business opportunities in the global functional food market.

In this chapter, we present a brief review of cultivation techniques, harvesting procedures and the geographical regions in China most favorable for premium wolfberry production.

Cultivation

The following section on cultivation was kindly provided by Ted Fogg and Amy Qi Lu who translated a Chinese paper on cultivation of a new wolfberry varietal named "NQ-1" by Zhang Shengyaun and colleagues of the Ningxia Research Institute, Yinchuan, China. This section, therefore, serves as an example of challenges and methods applied to successful cultivation of wolfberries.

NQ-1 is a new variety of wolfberry bred by the Ningxia Research Institute. It has particularly high yield and quality.

After four to eight years of field tests in various locations, NQ-1 was found to be 44% more productive than another varietal called "DaMaYe". Fruit weight of NQ-1 per one thousand berries exceeded that of DaMaYe by 21%. The *average* yield per year, as observed and calculated from 8 years after planting, is 161.4 kg of fruit. The yield specifically in the seventh year reached 274 kg. [Authors' note: yield is for 0.16 acre, a plot of land called a "mu" in Chinese].

Following are the cultivation skills gathered after several years of experiments and fieldwork on NQ-1.

Production of Healthy Nursery Stock

Site Preparation. The nursery should be a level lot located in an area of easy access, transport, efficient irrigation and drainage. The soil should be nutritious and of either sandy loam or light clay loam with approximate pH 8 and total salt under 0.2%.

Soil should be plowed to a depth 20 cm and be free of rocks and weeds. Application of 2500-5000 kg of mature manure per 1/6 acre was found effective. Divide the proposed site into 30-60 m^2 blocks with 4m long ditches and 1m wide ridges between every two ditches. Add 3 cm of fine sand onto the bed.

NQ-1 favors abundant sunlight, fertilizer, and moist conditions. It grows rapidly, branches abundantly, and has long, flexible shoots.

Nursery Stock Propagation. To insure the uniform quality of NQ-1 fruits, vegetation reproduction is used mainly from shoot cuttings.

Hardwood cutting: In late March—early April, before budding, select strong, well-nourished shoots with diameter 0.4 cm-0.6 cm and cut to 15 cm-20 cm long. Soak the cuttings in a rooting chemical for 24 hours. On the aforementioned ridge bed, insert cuttings into soil with 40 cm space between rows and 10 cm space within the row, leaving one or two buds on each cutting above ground, then mulch with a covering of plastic film.

Softwood cutting: In May-August, gather half-wooded shoots, cut them to 8-10 cm long, and remove the leaves below the middle of the cuttings. Then, apply a rooting chemical mixed with talc powder to the base of the cuttings. Insert cuttings 3 cm deep with 5 cm of spacing within the row and 10 cm between rows, then irrigate and cover with a plastic, arched tent to shade the cuttings.

Management During Growth of the Cutting. After the buds from hardwood cuttings have initiated sprouting, remove the ground film cover and keep the topsoil moist. During the initial 10-15 days after insertion of the softwood cuttings, mist the cuttings 2-3 times per day, and gradually reduce misting after this period. Once the young plant starts forming, slowly open the plastic tent to expose the plants. This aids their adaptation to the ambient environment. In early stages of stock growth, regularly irrigate and drain the excess water immediately. After irrigation, plow the soil and control weeds.

When new shoots from the hardwood cutting grow to 3-5 cm, keep only one strong shoot and thin out the rest. When this shoot grows to 60 cm, pinch the tip to control growth.

Bed Maintenance and Stock Preparation. Digging times are late March to early April or in autumn after leaves fall before freezing. While digging, avoid damaging roots and breaking shoots. After digging, immediately place the stock in a cool, shaded area and clear away damaged plants.

Stocks are graded into 3 categories depending on size: Grade 1 requires a height above 60 cm, diameter over 0.8 cm and more than 5 secondary roots, with a primary root of over 20 cm in length; Grade 2 has a height of 50-60 cm, diameter over 0.6 cm, 4 secondary roots, and a primary root of 15-20 cm; Grade 3 is determined by a height below 50 cm, diameter of about 0.5 cm, 2 to 4 secondary roots, and a primary root of 15-20 cm.

If stocks are not planted immediately, "heeling-in" must be conducted by choosing a high location (for good drainage) without direct wind exposure and checking regularly to avoid desiccation and rotting.

Orchard Establishment

Orchard Location. The orchard should have easy drainage and irrigation, ground water-table 1.5 m below the surface, total salt content below 0.2 %, pH about 8.0, and soil of sandy loam or light clay with deep subsoil.

Planting Blocks. Although the block size is determined by topography, the area should be around 1/6 acre.

Planting. Planting time is March to early April. Space between rows is 2-2.5 m. If machines are being used, the space should be 3-3.5 m. Spaces within a row are 1-1.5 m. Dig the holes in planned spots and add 2-3 kg of mature manure to each planting hole prior to planting.

Cultivation Practice

Soil Management and Weed Control. Shallowly cultivate the topsoil to a depth of 10-15 cm during early March to early April. During mid-months in May, June, and July, plow the topsoil to a depth of 6-10 cm to control weeds. From the middle of August to early September, till to a depth of 15-20 cm or shallower under a tree canopy.

Fertilizer Application

Organic Matter. In late October to early November, dig two symmetrical dressing furrows or one bend trench, both options requiring depth of 25-30 cm and width of 20-30 cm under the periphery of branches. This is needed to add organic manure (3000-3500 kg of aged animal manure) and 100 kg of by-products from food oil or 20 kg compound fertilizer per 1/6 acre. One to four year-old young trees should receive 1/3-1/2 of the total applications of the adult trees.

Compound fertilizers. Fertilizer is applied both to the soil and foliar.

Soil Addition. The total amount of added nitrogen should be divided into 3 applications. In late April, apply 14-15 kg of $CO(NH_2)2$ per 1/6 acre. In late May and June, apply 14-15 kg $(NH_4)2HPO_4$ per 1/6 acre.

Foliage dressing. Starting from late May through the entire blooming and bearing season, mist 150-200 kg of 0.5% compound-fertilizer (nitrogen, phosphorous, potassium (1:1:1)) to the tree canopy every 15-20 days per 1/6 acre.

Irrigation and Drainage. Water the orchard every 20-25 days during late April to middle June. Water every 15-20 days during late June to early August. Water 1-2 times during early September to late October. The first and last irrigations should be heavy ($60-80m^3$) per 1/6 acre. Light irrigation for growth season is appropriate. Excess water should be drained immediately.

Training and Pruning

Training Young Trees. Our goal is to form a sound framework to accelerate fruit bearing. In the first year, the central leader is determined by heading back the rooted cutting to 50-60 cm from the ground after planting. Select 3-5 strong side branches distributed evenly around the central leader as skeleton branches and cut these back to 10-20 cm to encourage secondary branching. Meanwhile, leave 3-4 side branches without topping on the central leader to become temporary bearing surfaces that encourage early fruiting. After the skeleton limbs have produced laterals, keep 1-2 of the laterals and cut these to 10 cm, allowing them to strengthen into minor scaffold branches.

In the second year, select one strong upward shoot from the underside of the scaffold limb as its extension. Head it back 10-20 cm to stimulate more shoots, then keep one or two shoots and head these back to 10 cm for bearing spurs. If there are any water shoots from the scaffold limbs or laterals, keep one and head it back 10-20 cm above the tree surface, then keep 4-5 of the secondary shootings to form the second-level bearing surface. Remove any branches coming off the leader branches.

During the third to fifth years, follow the procedure for Year 2 and use the leggy branches to fill and enlarge the canopy. If any straight-stand shoots rise from the uppermost region of central leader, keep one and head it back 10-20 cm above the tree surface. If no vertical shoots rise from central leader, choose 1-3 vertical shoots from the upper-level limbs within 15-20 cm of the central leader and head them back 20 cm above the tree surface.

After 5 years of training, trees average 1.6 m in height, 1.5 m in canopy diameter, and 6 cm in trunk diameter.

Pruning. The main focus of pruning is to rejuvenate the branches and establish a steady high-yielding plant. The principle is to remove all sprawling shoots, over crowded shoots, old week shoots, and root suckers. We want to cultivate vigorous shoots in empty spots of the canopy to produce new bearing spurs.

Spring pruning is conducted in middle-late April to remove dead branches (due to dehydration) from winter.

The goal of summer pruning is to remove nourishing shoots from the central leader or the major laterals. However, if the canopy has an opening or the leader's extension has died, keep the nourishing shoots and head them back to promote secondary shooting. In places without a leader, pinch out the vertical shoots to 10 cm higher than the surface of the canopy. In an empty spot, tipping height should be at the same level of the canopy and let secondary shoots develop into bearing spurs.

Winter pruning takes place after harvest or in February or March of the next year. Remove the strong shoots from the bottom and top of the central leader to regulate height of the tree. Thin out the old or weak branches inside the canopy. Remove any shoots that are old, weak, sprawling, vertical, infected (by pest or disease), overcrowded, or thorny.

Use strong shoots to fill the canopy by tipping to increase bearing surface and to extend the bearing period. Cut back overgrown branches or extra-large canopies. The lowest branches should be 30 cm above ground. After pruning, the shoots should be evenly spread and distributed for sunlight penetration and air circulation.

Harvesting and Drying Fruits

Harvest. The optimum harvest is when the fruit is 80%-90% ripe. Avoid harvesting after a rainfall. Berries require careful handling to avoid compression and bruising; one container should not exceed 10 kg wolfberries.

Drying. The two types are air seasoning and mechanical dehydration.

Air-seasoning—Spread the fresh berries 2 cm deep on an air exchange tray. Do not turn over the fruit before they are dry. Thump with a wooden stick on the bottom of the tray to accelerate the drying if extended rainy days are encountered.

Mechanical dehydration—Use hot air to blow dry. Put the berry-filled tray onto a trolley (one trolley for 10-16 trays). Deliver the trolley along the tracks into the drying facility. The drying facility has 3 temperature zones: the first zone is at 40-50 ° C (104-122° F) and berries are retained for 24 hours; the second zone has a temperature of 50-55 ° C (122-131° F) and berries stay 36-48 hours; and the third zone is at 55-65 ° C (131-149° F) and the berries remain for 24 hours. After over three days and three nights, the berries are taken out of the drying facility. Remove the stems and the berries are ready to be graded.

Disease and Pest Control

Integrated Control Method. Burn all infected branches and leaves and other field debris and eradicate any surrounding weeds. Strengthen irrigation and fertilization management to promote strong tree conditions.

Chemical Control. Depending on the condition of the disease or insect infection, choose appropriate chemicals, concentration of chemicals, and method of application as predetermined by the following table.

Table 10. Wolfberry plant pest control

Treatment	Disease or Pest	Method of Application
Dipterex (80% cream oil)	aphid, leaf miner, gall midge	800-1000x mist
Dimethoate(40% cream oil)	aphid, psylla, gall midge, gall mite, fruit moth, leaf miner	800-1000x mist
Tricresyl phosphate (50%)	Same as above	1000-1500x liquid mist onto canopy, 200x under canopy
Parathion (50% cream oil)	Same as above	1000x mist canopy 200x cover ground
Praponil (20%)	aphid, psylla, gall mite, rust mite	3000-4000x mist canopy
S emulsion (50%)	gall mite, rust mite, red spider	300x liquid mist
Trichoderma Powder (50%)	blackberry disease	600x mist
Carbendazine	gummosis	debark affected area, and brush concentration

Harvesting

The following section on harvesting was kindly provided by Ted Fogg and Amy Qi Lu who translated a Chinese paper on harvesting methods for wolfberries by Wang Xiling and colleagues of the Ningxia Research Institute, Yinchuan, China.

Optimum Fruit Picking Period

The wolfberry harvest season is very important to insure nutrient composition and the potential for health benefits from consuming wolfberries (Table 11; see also Chapter 10). Correctly using the optimum harvest period is essential for the quality and quantity of fruit. Also, the optimum harvest period is a main factor for increasing the commercial appeal of wolfberry fruit.

To discuss the optimum picking period, the following information is based on the different development stages of berries and the anticipated main nutrient contents of various stages.

Development Stages of the Ningxia Wolfberry

According to numerous observations of berry development, the berries need 35-40 days from blooming to fruit setting and ripening. Based on the berries' obvious color changes, the development stages can be classified into the following four stages: 1) young berry stage, 2) green berry stage, 3) color change stage, and 4) ripening stage. Details of each stage are discussed below with reference to the anatomical parts of the wolfberry plant.

- **Young berry stage.** From bloom to wilt of the corolla, the ovary is green-white and clearly enlarges. Inside the ovary, mitosis occurs and the mid-axel placenta yields multiple ovules. The initial endosperm forms.

- **Green berry stage.** The ovary changes from green-white to green. The berry extends from its calyx and the berry continues to enlarge until color starts to change. Now, the berry flesh is dense and the seeds are white while the pericarp is not dense. The endosperm is abundant and the ovary has become spherical.

- **Color change stage.** As the berry continues to develop, it changes from green to light greenish yellow to yellow-green to red-yellow to yellow-red. The fruit flesh is dense and the internal water content increases. The chlorophyll gradually disappears. The pericarp hardens and the endosperm is full. Meanwhile, the embryo leaves extend downward and are uneven in length.

- **Ripening stage.** The fruit both enlarges in size and ripens. The most characterized features of maturity are a bright red color (see front and back covers), softness and with optimum sweetness. Afterwards, the stem loosens and the fruits detach easily. The seeds are ripe, are a light yellow-white or light yellow-brown color, and are a flat, kidney shape. The seed coat stones. The mature embryo can now germinate.

Main Nutrient Contents at Each Development Stage of the Ningxia Wolfberry

According to a variety of chemical studies, wolfberries contain many kinds of organic materials including sugars, fats, proteins, amino acids, vitamins, polysaccharides, nucleotides, ash, water, and minerals [Authors' note: see Chapter 3].

The experimental berries for the data shown below are naturally dried berries with water content of 10-12%.

Essential organic materials related to fruit development

Some of the berry's inherent nutrients *decrease* during development from young berries to ripe berries; these include total amino acids, raw proteins, total nitrogen, calcium, phosphorus, and betaine.

Other of the berry's inherent nutrients *increase or remain stable* from young berries to ripe berries; these include beta-carotene, vitamins B1, B2 and C and iron. The total sugar content increases progressively over 3-fold from color change stage to early ripening. This change gives fresh wolfberries their special sweet taste.

Early ripening and ripening stages. Betaine, raw protein, total nitrogen, vitamins B1 and B2 and beta-carotene all show significant decreases by over 20% while calcium and phosphorus decrease by about 15%. Only vitamin C content significantly increases by about 50% during this stage. Iron increases by about 13%. Total amino acid and total sugar contents increase by 5%.

Therefore, to preserve berry quality, optimal harvest for taste should be brought forward to the early ripening stage.

Using Color of Dried Berries to Estimate Optimal Harvest Time

The fresh wolfberry fruit is a berry with thin skin and abundant juice having water content of about 80%. Only after dehydration can berries become commercial products suitable for shipping and storage.

Two methods of dehydration are to dry directly in the sun or to force-dry with a commercial blower. In Ningxia, old production areas and individual producers mainly use natural dehydration methods relying on sunlight. Large farms may use hot air blowers for dehydration.

When drying conditions are the same but harvest maturities are different, both drying methods produce dried berries that have different surface colors according to stage of maturity. If the fruits are picked during the late color change stage or the early ripening stage, the dried fruits are bright red (e.g., see back cover).

If the fruits are picked at the ripe stage, the dried fruits are red, dark red, violet red, blackish red, or brownish red. This color variation is due to the pigment content and sugar content at harvest. Fruits picked during the early color change stage dry to a light red color. This is due to reduced pigment and sugar content.

The optimum picking period should be during the early ripening stage or the late color change stage. Detailed harvest indicators and berry characteristics:

- **Berry exterior characteristics.** A bright red color and a shiny

pericarp are the outstanding indicators for the early ripening
stage.
- **Berry seed characteristics.** The seed coat has changed from
  white to yellow-white or light yellow-brown and has ossified.

Picking Technique

To insure berry quality, harvest should be conducted on clear, bright
mornings or evenings. Avoid harvest during times in early morning when
the dew is still prevalent, after rain and in hot sun, as these conditions
decrease berry quality.

Fresh wolfberries are delicate and vulnerable to bruising, squashing
and compression damage. Therefore, during harvest, pick carefully and
place lightly into trays. Containers should hold less than 10 kg of weight
to avoid damaging the bottom fruit.

Table 11. Nutrient analysis during wolfberry development stages

Nutrient	Young Berry Stage	Green Berry Stage	Color Change Stage	Early Ripening Stage	Ripe Stage	% Change, Early Ripe to Ripe Stage
Total Sugar, %	3.8	3.2	16.3	52.5	54.8	+ 4
Protein, %	25.7	25.3	22.1	14.5	11.5	- 21
Total Nitrogen, %	4.1	4.1	3.6	2.3	1.8	- 22
Total Amino Acids, mg/100g	16.9	16.8	13.4	8.5	9.0	+ 6
Calcium, mg/100g	170	154	109	87	73	- 16
Iron, mg/100g	9	9	12	8	9	+ 13
Phosphorus, mg/100g	433	481	392	268	222	- 17
Vitamin B_1, mg/100g	0.17	0.20	0.14	0.21	0.15	- 29
Vitamin B_2, mg/100g	1.2	2.0	1.5	1.8	1.4	- 22
Vitamin C, mg/100g	Trace	1.6	11.9	12.4	18.4	+ 48
Beta-carotene, mg/100g	0.2	0.3	13.0	11.5	8.3	- 28

Table Summary. From this analysis by wolfberry crop scientists in Ningxia, it is clear that nutrient quality changes considerably as ripening of the fruit occurs. As wolfberries are usually consumed fresh or prepared for drying from ripe fruit, the ripe stage is a focus at which time the wolfberries have

- *The highest brix or sugar content {Authors' note: measured at 26 brix units, Chapter 3}*
- *Reduced protein concentration (probably due to the higher water content at this stage)*
- *Lower concentration of several vitamins, minerals and the carotenoid, beta-carotene (Authors' note: likely due to an increase in the amount of juice)*
- *Higher vitamin C content {Authors' note: measured at 29 mg per 100 g dried fruit, Chapter 3}*

[end of translated section]

Effect of Modern Agricultural Practices

It is not known precisely to what extent changes in crop management and soil conditions affect the nutrient quality of today's wolfberries in China. Evidence from other studies, however, gives clear indication for concern that pressures for growing more wolfberries on the same plot of land, as has occurred for strawberries and other fruit crops, could diminish nutrient density.

A senior executive of a berry extract firm in the US was quoted as saying,

"When food scientists analyzed fruits and vegetables grown in the 1950s and compared them to the same crops in 1999, they found lower levels of key nutrients like vitamin C, calcium, iron, and phytochemicals."

"While farmers in the *1950s produced four tons* of strawberries per acre, *today's farmers, using fungicides and other chemicals, produce 40 tons of berries from the same land.* It only makes sense that when a plant yields a 10-fold increase in fruit, the nutritive value can be compromised."

Even with this concern, Ningxia's agricultural productivity is exceptional, sometimes attributed with 2-4 times the crop yields (due to greater soil fertility) compared to other China regions. It is likely that annual flooding by the Huang He provides renewal of fertile loess deposited as river sediment over Ningxia's wolfberry fields.

Consequently, as the economy for wolfberries grows in future years, these factors will need to be taken into account to maintain and promote the fruit's extraordinary nutrient quality and popular taste.

Main Geographical Regions

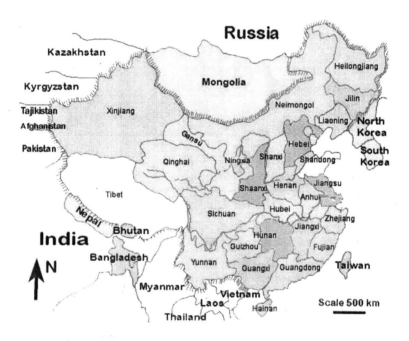

Map of China. The Huang He (Yellow River) originates in Xinjiang (western boundary) and courses eastward through main regions of wolfberry growing, including Ningxia (center), China's most famous province for wolfberries.

As inferred in Chapter 8, the Chinese autonomous regions of Ningxia and Xinjiang have been famous for wolfberries over centuries. In this chapter, we want to present brief discussions of these geographic regions to highlight soil and climatic factors that could be important for wolfberry nutrient content.

Typical of produce-rich areas in many parts of the world, soil favorable for high-quality wolfberry growth in China is found mainly along river plains where nutrients renew annually from the processes of erosion, floods and weather.

Ningxia

As China's largest river system, the Huang He (Yellow River) region and its tributaries, flood plains, valleys and banks passing through Ningxia are where the densest and most prized crops of wolfberries now grow.

The Huang He travels a total of 5464 km, much of this distance over arid infertile lands in western China before reaching Gansu Province west of the Ningxia region. It is believed that Gansu's soils wind-eroding into the Huang He affect the sediment conditions along the Huang He banks downstream in Ningxia.

When the Huang He floods as it has done over millennia, deep mineral-rich silt settles across its riverside plains, providing nourishment for a diversity of managed and wild crops. This beneficial soil condition is the effect created mainly by the Loess Plateau in Gansu through which the Huang He flows before reaching the Ningxia wolfberry fields.

Finer than sand, yellow Gansu loess was formed 2 million years ago after glaciation left behind mineral dust that has been wind-eroded into the Huang He ever since. Gansu erosion is so dense that silt content in the Huang He weighs *35 kg for every cubic meter of water*—the most silt-laden river water on Earth.

In Ningxia, the Huang He silt after flooding becomes a nutrient-rich soil unique in the world and almost certainly a foundation for wolfberries to synthesize their rich contents of nutrients.

The beautiful Ningxia region, named after "xia" meaning "peaceful summer", is called China's *Herbal Medicine Valley* renowned for the country's premium agricultural products. Organic-grade quality common in Ningxia earns certificates for the prestigious "Green Status" from the Chinese Ministry of Health, similar to an organic certification in the United States.

So popular are Ningxia wolfberries that there is an annual wolfberry festival, held in Xinhua in mid-August each year, an internationally-recognized statue tribute to wolfberry harvesting in the town and numerous local legends of long-term health benefits to Ningxia residents eating wolfberries over their lives.

Background provided in the book by Mindell and Handel is worth repeating here. One story from the Tang Dynastry poet Liu Yuxi (722-802 AD) gives account of a Ningxia water well into which wolfberries had been falling for centuries. Those who drank the water gained a lifelong bounty of nutrients from this wolfberry (goji) water.

The Goji Well
(Liu Yuxi, Tang Dynasty, circa 800 AD)

A cool well beside the monk's house,
A clear spring feeds the well and water has great powers.
Emerald green leaves grow on the wall,
The deep red berries shine like copper,
The flourishing branch like a walking stick,
The old root in a dog's shape signals good fortune.
The goji nourishes body and spirit.
Drink of the well and enjoy a long life.

With a geographical area of 66,000 sq. km, population of about 6 million (2005 est.) and capital city of Yinchuan, Ningxia is situated in the north-central part of China at the Great Bend of the Huang He (above map). It is surrounded in the west and north by Inner Mongolia while the southern and eastern regions are bounded by Gansu Province and Shanxi Province, respectively. Gansu contains regions of the Loess Plateau, the highly erodible wastelands that contribute mineral-rich silt into the Huang He affecting the downstream plains and cultivated wolfberry fields of Ningxia.

Ningixa's altitude averages about 2000 meters, having a climate of cold/wet in the south and warm/dry in the north bordered by the Tengger, Maowusu, and Ulan Buh deserts.

Ningxia's climate has summer daytime temperatures rising to as high as 39 °C and those in winter plummeting to as low as 30 °C below zero. The day\night temperature variation in summer averages 17°, thought by horticulturalists to be good for crops to synthesize starch such as the high polysaccharide content (sweetness) of Ningxia wolfberries.

Ningxia has over a million acres of river basin and wasteland suitable for farming. There are 3 million acres of exploitable meadows, making Ningxia a major pasture and crop region of China. The Wuyin Plain of northern Ningxia consists of land irrigated with water diverted from the Huang He whose annual irrigation for farming purposes has been estimated at 32.5 billion cubic meters.

The rich land resources, convenient irrigation conditions to divert water from the Huang He, and abundant sunshine in the north create an ideal foundation for Ningxia wolfberry agriculture.

Other fruit crops such as watermelons, apples, and grapes have a 20 percent higher sugar content than those produced in central China. These same factors may impart desirable qualities for wolfberries. High juice content (80% or greater water content in ripe fruit), premium sweetness (high brix of about 26, Chapter 3) and legendary health benefits are renowned characteristics of the highest grade Ningxia wolfberries.

Over centuries, according to Mindell and Handel, Chinese provinces other than Ningxia or Xinjiang have claimed the title as wolfberry's best growing region—Hebei, Gansu, Qinghai, Shanxi, Changshan, and Shandong (Mindell and Handel map, p 21).

Several factors are offered in their book as support for wolfberry growing requirements to form the most premium berries, such as an alkaline soil (pH around 8.2) and an annual temperature range of 102 °F to-16 °F (38.5 °C to-27 °C).

Further focus by Mindell and Handel is on the wolfberry polysaccharides as a signature nutrient class that can be analyzed by spectral methods to help define where the best wolfberries are grown (Chapter 8), i.e., more polysaccharide richness equates to better wolfberries. This may be a traceable characteristic according to geography and spectral signature. Mindell and Handel discuss that Ningxia, Xinjiang and Himalaya berries have the best spectra and are similar in exceptional polysaccharide content.

These spectral studies are interesting preliminary data but remain hypotheses that have not been published under peer-review nor have they been confirmed by other scientific reports to date.

Xinjiang

Of potential interest, although not well-documented by independent research, is the claim by Mindell and Handel that Himalayan oases and valleys of Xinjiang Autonomous Region in western China, bordering Kyrgyzstan and Kazakhstan (map), are the best growing regions for wolfberries. Runoff from mountain streams and soil residue from millennia of earthquakes and land upheavals as the Tianshan and Himalayan Mountains formed may have created unusually nutrient-rich soils especially favorable for growing nutrient-dense wolfberries.

There is also some speculation that high altitude (plateaus are 2,000-5,000 m), extreme annual weather changes, large diurnal temperature range during growing season, mountain water and soil characteristics combine to challenge biochemical defenses that become constituted in the berries and so make Xinjiang wolfberries unique for high nutrient density. This is a fascinating area deserving of further plant research.

Mindell and Handel claim there are 18,440 species of plants in Xinjiang, many unique only to this region of the world. Over 8,000 of these plants are thought by traditional herbal practitioners to have medicinal properties.

Xinjiang is China's largest autonomous province, having a surface area of 1.66 million square kilometers and occupying one-sixth of China's national territory. Xinjiang has lengthy borders of which 5,400 km contact eight foreign countries. With a population 1 6 million, Xinjiang has Urumqi as its capital.

Surrounded by mountains supplying snowmelt for irrigation, Xinjiang's agricultural territories account for much of its economy. To harness the supply of melt, rivers have been rechanneled into irrigation canals over hundreds of years, now providing Xinjiang with some 400 reservoirs and 30,000 km of developed irrigation. Despite these favorable resources for agriculture, however, much of the vast Xinjiang region is infertile desert.

Summary

Although there is an intriguing long history of wolfberry farming in many regions of China, it now seems clear that this plant can grow almost anywhere in different climates.

It is perhaps the unique soil conditions created by loessal silt deposited on the Huang He flood plains that contribute to premium nutrient and taste quality of Ningxia wolfberries. Xinjiang and the valleys of the Himalayas in western China have also been purported to have high quality wolfberries, although no objective evidence exists for this distribution.

Soil conditions, irrigation, weather, altitude factors, favorable propagation methods, lack of persistent pests, human cultivation methods and phytogenetics likely combine to afford central-western China with ideal growing conditions assuring premium wolfberries.

One need only consider these factors as similar to those for grapes in the more familiar industry of wine making, i.e., numerous local soil, weather, irrigation, cultivating, genetic and processing factors converge to determine differences in quality of two similar wines, even between adjacent vineyards in the same grape-growing region.

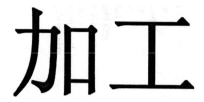

加工

CHAPTER 10
Processing Effects on Wolfberry Nutrients

As with any fruit, wolfberries can be processed into a variety of raw materials for dietary, functional food or beverage applications. Fresh or dried berries, juice, whole berry pulp or pomace, puree, powders of juice or pomace, seed powder and oils, leaves, bark, roots, extracts (such as individual carotenoids or pigments for coloring) from any plant component are some of the raw materials of interest for product development.

As our core interest in this book has been to present the nutrient quality of wolfberries, we can ask whether the usual steps of processing affect nutrient content. There has been no scientific work specifically on the effects of wolfberry processing to give us a foundation for this critical area affecting nutritional quality. Considerable study of processing methods on other berries and fruit, however, allows us to extrapolate possible effects on wolfberry nutrients.

With this as an understanding, we have to treat the material of this chapter as speculative at best while awaiting more specific wolfberry research in the future.

Of principal concern is that fruit undergoing any type of processing or storage might have its nutrients altered in uncertain amounts, even in the earliest procedures after harvesting when delicate fruit is machine-handled for inspection (picture below).

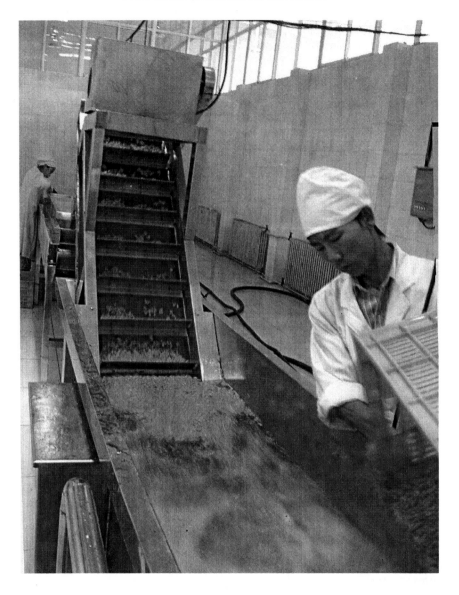

Post-harvest screening of wolfberries on Rich Nature's farm, Ningxia, China.

Breeding, cultivation and processing procedures may collectively be significant factors affecting variation of nutrients found in fruit and vegetables, yet breeders and processors do not yet work together routinely to ensure optimum levels of healthy compounds.

This is perhaps due to the lack of scientific and consumer awareness—

and therefore demand—for information on particular fruit and vegetable nutrients.

One ancillary but important bearing on this issue is the ability to compare scientific data on nutrients of a given plant studied and reported by different research groups. If processing of the plant samples between laboratories has been significantly different, then data on nutrients may be artifactually affected, leading to confusion about actual contents.

Consequently, this is an important area of future research on wolfberry raw materials to understand processing factors to prepare fruit for further scientific analyses and for export from China or any origin over long shipping distances and storage durations for further processing.

To gain some grasp of these issues, we reviewed relevant literature about the effects of processing on berries more thoroughly studied to date, then summarized in this chapter how wolfberry nutrients may fare under similar treatment.

Our review indicates that berry processing has considerable effect on the nutritional and phytochemical properties of fruit, casting caution toward interpretation of nutrients remaining and in what amounts. Important categories concerning nutrient density and quality are

A. Interspecies and berry plant component variation
B. Berry growing or ripening characteristics
C. Methods for berry storage: Preparation and storage variables
D. Effects of temperature on processing and storage of berries

A. Interspecies and plant component variation

1. Kalt W, Ryan DA, Duy JC, Prior RL, Ehlenfeldt MK, Vander Kloet SP. Agriculture and Agri-Food Canada, Kentville, Nova Scotia B4N 1J5, Canada. **Interspecies variation in anthocyanins, phenolics, and antioxidant capacity among genotypes of highbush and lowbush blueberries (Vaccinium section cyanococcus spp.).** J Agric Food Chem. 2001 Oct;49(10):4761-7.

In this well-known study, Kalt and coworkers showed that popular blueberry species—the lowbush wild blueberry and highbush cultivated blueberry—differed in contents of antioxidant phytochemicals (anthocyanins and phenolic acids) and vitamin C, the lowbush specie having higher values. Also, blueberries had much higher contents of anthocyanins than strawberries or raspberries which, by contrast, had higher vitamin C contents than blueberries. Vitamin C made only a minor

(<9%) contribution to the overall antioxidant capacity of these berries. Storage for 8 days at temperatures above freezing actually increased the antioxidant capacities of strawberries and raspberries.

The study results may apply to differences in antioxidant and vitamin C contents between wolfberry species and to changes in antioxidant capacity during cold storage. In other words, species variation among wolfberries may readily account for differences in nutrient content of berries from similar geographical regions.

2. Kalt W, Forney CF, Martin A, Prior RL. Agriculture and Agri-Food Canada, Atlantic Food and Horticulture Research Centre, Kentville, Nova Scotia, Canada. **Antioxidant capacity, vitamin C, phenolics, and anthocyanins after fresh storage of small fruits.** J Agric Food Chem. 1999 Nov;47(11):4638-44.

This study showed that wild lowbush blueberries had higher antioxidant capacity (higher concentration of anthocyanins and phenolic acids) than cultivated highbush blueberries. As wild blueberries are smaller in size than their highbush cousins, additional tests were performed to analyze whether physical size of a berry actually influenced antioxidant content—it did not in this study, although other research since this publication has concluded that berry skin antioxidants per gram must be more concentrated in smaller berries since the ratio of skin to pulp surface area is greater in small fruits.

The method of extraction influenced the composition of berry extracts; the highest anthocyanin, total phenolic contents and antioxidant capacity were found in extracts obtained using methanol as the solvent.

For wolfberries, this study may indicate that size differences among berries of different Lycium barbarum cultivars probably do not account for any nutrient variation. There are, however, opposite conclusions from different research (Chapter 9).

3. Ehlenfeldt MK, Prior RL. Marucci Center for Blueberry and Cranberry Research and Extension, Agricultural Research Service, U.S. Department of Agriculture, Chatsworth, NJ, USA **Oxygen radical absorbance capacity (ORAC) and phenolic and anthocyanin concentrations in fruit and leaf tissues of highbush blueberry.** J Agric Food Chem. 2001 May;49(5):2222-7.

This extensive study of 87 varietals of highbush blueberries for both their fruit and leaves showed the interesting result that leaves actually have higher antioxidant capacity than berries.

Tea from wolfberry leaves has been used as an herbal drink in China for thousands of years. If these results from blueberries apply to wolfberries, then tea and other beverage or food applications using wolfberry leaves may prove of interest for gaining antioxidant benefits in functional beverages.

4. Rimando AM, Kalt W, Magee JB, Dewey J, Ballington JR. Natural Products Utilization Research Unit, ARS, US Department of Agriculture, University, MS, USA, Agriculture and Agri-Food Canada, Kentville, Nova Scotia, Canada. **Resveratrol, pterostilbene, and piceatannol in vaccinium berries.** J Agric Food Chem. 2004 Jul 28;52(15):4713-9.

This analysis of antioxidant chemicals in cultivars of 10 blueberry species from different geographic regions indicated that particularly resveratrol—the beneficial phenolic antioxidant commonly linked to red grapes and wine—varied between species.

Wolfberry nutrients also likely vary in nutrient density between species and regions of China where it grows.

5. Gil MI, Tomas-Barberan FA, Hess-Pierce B, Holcroft DM, Kader AA. Department of Pomology, University of California, Davis, CA, USA; **Antioxidant activity of pomegranate juice and its relationship with phenolic composition and processing.** J Agric Food Chem. 2000 Oct;48(10):4581-9.

This study examined antioxidant chemicals in pomegranate juice made from arils (pulp-like covering over seeds) plus rind or just arils alone. The activity was higher in commercial juices extracted from whole pomegranates that included the rind compared to experimental juices obtained only from arils. This shows that pomegranate industrial processing extracts some of the antioxidants present in the fruit rind, a valuable source of nutrients. Multiple antioxidants, including anthocyanins, ellagic acid derivatives, and tannins were detected and quantified in the pomegranate juices.

The results raise a question important for considering nutrient sources *within* a plant independently or together. Different segments of the wolfberry plant, e.g., its pulp, seeds, skin and leaves, may each contribute valuable phytochemicals and nutrients. Thus, a stronger antioxidant capacity likely results from a wolfberry preparation that includes skin and seeds.

The wolfberry juice called NingXia Red is made from a puree of the wolfberry fruit including its skin and stem, likely contributing stronger phytochemical composition and antioxidant quality than its predecessor, Berry Young Juice.

6. Tsao R, Yang R, Xie S, Sockovie E, Khanizader S. Food Research Program, Agriculture and Agri-Food Canada, Guelph, Ontario, Canada. **Which polyphenolic compounds contribute to the total antioxidant capacities of apples?** J Agric Food Chem, 2005 Jun 15;53(12):4989-95.

Although there was considerable detail in this study of apples, a main finding perhaps relevant to wolfberries and other fruits was that peel (i.e., skin) had much greater antioxidant concentrations than pulp. This finding provides another example of whole food nutritional value in diets when compared to extract supplements, fruit flesh only or juices. Simply stated, eating the skin of fruits provides phytochemicals potentially valuable for health.

B. Berry growing or ripening characteristics

Already introduced in Table 11, Chapter 9 was evidence that nutrient content of the wolfberry changes as the fruit ripens, a process sometimes called "maturation" or "development". Of particular note for one of wolfberry's main antioxidant nutrients, vitamin C (ascorbic acid), its content *increased* substantially from the green berry stage (1.6 mg/100 g) to the early ripening and fully ripe stages where vitamin C content became maximal (12-18 mg/100 g).

Accordingly, we give special attention below to the development or ripening effects on nutrient content of wolfberries by drawing inferences from studies on other berries.

7. Raffo, A, Paoletti, F, Antonelli, M. **Changes in sugar, organic acid, flavonol and carotenoid composition during ripening of berries of three seabuckthorn (*Hippophae rhamnoides* L.) cultivars,** Euro Food Res Technol 2004, 219(4); 360-8.

This study on seabuckthorn berry cultivars showed that vitamin C levels decreased progressively during ripening and carotenoid (beta-carotene, zeaxanthin, beta-cryptoxanthin) contents increased over the ripening period. Overall, harvesting dates were important in determining when nutrient densities were greatest.

Wolfberries likely display similar variations in nutrient content over the durations of berry maturation on the vine (see Table 11, Chapter 9). As wolfberry carotenoids are of significant antioxidant interest, we may tentatively conclude that late-harvest wolfberries yield the highest contents of carotenoids and so may afford the greatest antioxidant value.

8. Piland D, Howard LR, Cho MJ, Clark JR, Department of Food Science, University of Arkansas, Fayetteville, AR. **Antioxidant capacity and phenolic content of bluecrop and ozarkblue blueberries as affected by maturation,** International Food Technologies Annual Meeting 2003—meeting presentation, http://ift.confex.com/ift/2003/techprogram/paper_17794.htm

This interesting research explored whether antioxidant capacity in blueberries varied according to when the berries were harvested. Levels of ORAC, total phenolics and hydroxycinnamates generally decreased from the green stage of early ripening to 75% blue stages of maturity and then increased from 75% blue to 100% blue stages of maturity. Total anthocyanin content increased from the green stage to the 100% blue stage of maturity, with the largest increase occurring from 75% to 100% blue stages of maturity. Flavonol content decreased from green to the 100% blue stage of maturity.

Phytonutrient content of wolfberries no doubt is complex, having many factors affecting it over the course of maturation on the vine (Table 11, Chapter 9). Simply with stage of ripening, the above research shows that time of harvesting is important for fixing the antioxidant content in berries. Highest overall antioxidant content possibly occurs when the wolfberry fruit is reddest in color and most mature on the vine. These factors have potential commercial importance if maximizing ORAC in wolfberries was a desired characteristic for commercial growers and food processors.

Further recent research (abstract below) on ripening of cherries showed that the antioxidants, phenolics, anthocyanins and vitamin C, peaked in concentration at a time when skin color began to darken.

9. Serrano M, Guillen F, Martinez-Romero D, Castillo S, Valero D. Department of Applied Biology and Department of Food Technology, EPSO, University Miguel Hernandez, Alicante, Spain. **Chemical**

constituents and antioxidant activity of sweet cherry at different ripening stages. J Agric Food Chem. 2005 Apr 6;53(7):2741-5.

The development and ripening process of sweet cherry (Prunus avium L. cv. 4-70) on the tree was evaluated. For this purpose, 14 different stages were selected in accordance with homogeneous size and color. Some parameters related to fruit quality, such as color, texture, sugars, organic acids, total antioxidant activity, total phenolic compounds, anthocyanins, and ascorbic acid were analyzed. The results revealed that in sweet cherry, the changes in skin color, glucose and fructose accumulation, and softening process are initiated at early developmental stages, coinciding with the fast increase in fruit size. Also, the decrease in color parameter was correlated with the greatest accumulation of total anthocyanins. Ascorbic acid, total antioxidant activity (TAA), and total phenolic compounds decreased during the early stages of sweet cherry development but exponentially increased from stage 8, which coincided with the anthocyanin accumulation and fruit darkening. TAA showed positive correlations (r = 0.99) with both ascorbic acid and total phenolic compounds and also with the anthocyanin concentration from stage 8.

In another study of antioxidant phytochemical changes during ripening, the authors found that raspberries produced new antioxidants as the fruit ripened (Beekwilder et al., 2005, see references); in other words, part of the ripening process is to make new phytochemicals having potential health benefits both for the plant itself and to animals that consume the fruit.

Beekwilder and colleagues concluded that antioxidant content (or perhaps measurements of ORAC) could be used as a quality parameter of berry fruit during ripening. This is a novel and useful consideration for employing the ORAC measurement on food labels as an index both of antioxidant intensity and ripeness.

C. Methods for berry storage: Preparation and storage variables

10. Connor AM, Luby JJ, Hancock JF, Berkheimer S, Hanson EJ. Department of Horticultural Science, University of Minnesota, St. Paul, Minnesota 55108, **Changes in fruit antioxidant activity among blueberry cultivars during cold-temperature storage,** J Agric Food Chem. 2002 Feb 13;50(4):893-8.

During the time they retained marketable quality, one cultivar of blueberry demonstrated a 29% increase in antioxidant activity, but no cultivars showed a decrease from the harvest antioxidant activity value during storage at 5 °C.

This study demonstrated that increases in antioxidant activity, total phenolic content, and anthocyanin content may occur in the blueberry during cold storage and are cultivar-dependent. Wolfberries cold-stored and of different species may similarly show subtle changes in antioxidant activity.

11. Lohachoompol V, Srzednicki G, Craske J. **The change of total anthocyanins in blueberries and their antioxidant effect after drying and freezing.** J Biomed Biotechnol. 2004;(5):248-252

The main finding of this study was that frozen highbush blueberries did not show any significant decrease in anthocyanin levels during three months of storage. As a test of drying methods, osmotic treatment to dehydrate the berries followed by thermal treatment produced greater reduction of anthocyanins than thermal treatment alone.

12. Zheng Y, Wang CY, Wang SY, Zheng W. Produce Quality and Safety Laboratory and Fruit Laboratory, Beltsville Agricultural Research Center, U.S. Department of Agriculture, Beltsville, Maryland, USA. **Effect of high-oxygen atmospheres on blueberry phenolics, anthocyanins, and antioxidant capacity.** J Agric Food Chem. 2003 Nov 19;51(24):7162-9.

This research showed that elevated oxygen levels between 60 and 100% increased total phenolics and total anthocyanins in blueberries under storage conditions. Fruit treated with oxygen concentrations above 60% exhibited significantly less decay in storage, demonstrating overall that treatment of berries with high-oxygen concentrations may preserve antioxidant capacity during periods of storage.

13. Asami DK, Hong YJ, Barrett DM, Mitchell AE. Department of Food Science and Technology, University of California-Davis, USA. **Comparison of the total phenolic and ascorbic acid content of freeze-dried and air-dried marionberry, strawberry, and corn grown using conventional, organic, and sustainable agricultural practices.** J Agric Food Chem. 2003 Feb 26;51(5):1237-41.

This study showed that freeze-drying preserved higher levels of total phenolics of berries in comparison with air-drying. Although more expensive, freeze-drying may be important to some wolfberry producers for preserving phytochemical value during long-term storage.

In more recent studies on drying effects, Rababah and coworkers (2005, references) showed that dehydration increased ORAC and the concentration of anthocyanins and phenolics in strawberries. Although a practical issue for reporting concentrations, this analysis shows that dried preparations are likely to have higher concentrations when expressed per weight of berry fruit.

14. Wu X, Beecher GR, Holden JM, Haytowitz DB, Gebhardt SE, Prior RL. Arkansas Children's Nutrition Center and Agricultural Research Service, U.S. Department of Agriculture, Little Rock, Arkansas, USA. **Lipophilic and hydrophilic antioxidant capacities of common foods in the United States.** J Agric Food Chem. 2004 Jun 16;52(12):4026-37.

Although the main goal of this study was to define oxygen radical absorbance capacities (ORAC), i.e., antioxidant capacities, of numerous fruits and vegetables, an ancillary analysis was to evaluate the effects of food processing as it affects ORAC.

Removal of peel from apples lowered ORAC (see 2005 study on apples by Tsao et al., above). Cooking (baking, boiling) increased ORAC in some species such as potatoes and tomatoes (Solanaceae plant family relatives of wolfberry), presumably by liberating antioxidant phytochemicals from skin, whereas cooking lowered ORAC in broccoli and carrots (foods without skin). Although these analyses were not complete, they indicate variable effects of cooking on phytochemicals probably relevant to wolfberry processing and thus in need of systematic research.

The public media has provided a relevant example particularly for gaining the benefits of lycopenes from processed tomatoes. For example, using tomato sauces or ketchup gives higher lycopene intake values than eating raw tomatoes. Although speculation, this finding may mean that the carotenoids in wolfberries, primarily beta-carotene and zeaxanthin, may be more bioavailable in cooked or processed wolfberries. Some have discussed this effect as resulting from the liberation of carotenoids from the skin of tomatoes during the maceration process in sauce or ketchup production.

Although not specifically analyzed, other variables affecting ORAC were discussed by these authors, including seasonal effects of climate and weather, genetics, growing environment, pest exposure, diseases, etc. All these factors would need to be controlled or isolated to determine the precise impact of processing on wolfberry nutrients.

An additional value of these studies is to show that ORAC is a simple measure that reflects overall quality and possible degrading effects on berry fruit.

Quite possibly in the near future, food labels will use ORAC as an index of how carefully fruit and other fresh foods have been processed or stored.

15. Boyer J, Liu RH, Department of Food Science and Institute of Comparative and Environmental Toxicology, Cornell University, Ithaca, New York, **Apple phytochemicals and their health benefits,** Nutr J 2004, 3:5

Because apple peels contain more antioxidant compounds, especially the flavonoid quercetin, apple peels may have higher antioxidant activity and higher bioactivity than apple flesh. Research showed that apples without peels had less antioxidant activity than apples with peels. Apples with peels have been shown to better inhibit cancer cell proliferation when compared to apples without peels. Apple peels contain 2-6x (depending on the variety) more phenolic compounds than flesh, and 2-3x more flavonoids than flesh.

For antioxidant-rich wolfberries, this review indicates that whole fruit containing skin and seeds, or pomace from whole berries, would have more phytochemicals present than in juice.

D. Effects of temperature on processing and storage

16. Gahler S, Otto K, Bohm V. Institute of Nutrition, Friedrich Schiller University Jena, Germany. **Alterations of vitamin C, total phenolics, and antioxidant capacity as affected by processing tomatoes to different products.** J Agric Food Chem. 2003 Dec 31;51(27):7962-8.

As a relative of the wolfberry, tomatoes and the various ways they are processed offer insights to preserving nutrients during different processing steps toward juice, sauce or soup. The vitamin C contents of the tomato products decreased during the thermal processing of tomatoes into juice, sauce and soup. In contrast, total phenolics concentration and water soluble antioxidant capacity increased during these steps. A primary carotenoid antioxidant of tomatoes, lycopene, is known from this study to become more bioavailable when tomatoes are processed into juice or sauce, probably because it is released from skin (above discussion and paper #6).

Accordingly, we might expect wolfberry's nutrients, especially its carotenoids, to show similar outcomes from processing. Vitamin C content may be reduced by processing and carotenoid antioxidants increased.

17. Hakkinen SH, Karenlampi SO, Mykkanen HM, Torronen AR. Department of Clinical Nutrition, Department of Physiology, University of Kuopio, Finland. **Influence of domestic processing and storage on flavonol contents in berries.** J Agric Food Chem. 2000 Jul;48(7):2960-5.

This study is valuable because it examined the fate of antioxidant phytochemicals during common domestic production of jam or juice from different berries. Cooking strawberries with sugar to make jam resulted in minor losses of the antioxidant flavonoids, quercetin 15% and kaempferol 18%. During cooking of bilberries with water and sugar to make soup, 40% of quercetin was lost. Traditional preservation of crushed lingonberries in their own juice caused a considerable (40%) loss of quercetin.

Only 15% of quercetin and 30% of myricetin present in unprocessed berries were retained in juices made by common domestic methods (steam-extracted blackcurrant juice, unpasteurized lingonberry juice). Cold-pressing was superior to steam-extraction in extracting flavonols from blackcurrants. During 9 months of storage at 20 C, quercetin content decreased markedly (40%) in bilberries and lingonberries, but not in blackcurrants or red raspberries. Myricetin and kaempferol were more susceptible than quercetin to losses during storage.

Although these same phenolic flavonols have not been demonstrated in wolfberries, the overall results indicate that processing into common domestic products like jam or juice diminishes berry antioxidants.

18. Lyons MM, Yu C, Toma RB, Cho SY, Reiboldt W, Lee J, van Breemen RB. Food and Nutritional Science Division, California State University-Long Beach, Long Beach, CA, USA. **Resveratrol in raw and baked blueberries and bilberries.** J Agric Food Chem. 2003 Sep 24;51(20):5867-70.

Mentioned above, resveratrol is the antioxidant phenolic most commonly associated with health benefits in red grapes and wine. This study examined its fate in 4 species of blueberry during baking.

Because blueberries and bilberries are often consumed after cooking, the effect of baking on resveratrol content was studied after 18 min of heating at 190 degrees C. Seventeen to 46% of the resveratrol degraded in the various Vaccinium species from this short duration heating. Therefore, resveratrol content of baked or heat-processed blueberries or bilberries should be expected to be lower than in raw fruit. Although blueberries and bilberries were found to contain resveratrol, the level of this valued antioxidant in these fruits was <10% that reported for fresh red grapes. Thus, cooking or heat processing of berries contributes to degradation of resveratrol.

We are unaware of analyses for resveratrol in wolfberries. Nevertheless, this study indicates that heat processing of berries for domestic uses is likely to degrade antioxidant qualities in wolfberries.

19. Kaack K, Austed T. Department of Food Science and Technology, Aarslev, Denmark. **Interaction of vitamin C and flavonoids in elderberry (Sambucus nigra L.) during juice processing.** Plant Foods Hum Nutr. 1998;52(3):187-98.

This interesting study tested the effects of ascorbic acid content (vitamin C) and presence of oxygen on the phytonutrient antioxidants, quercetin and anthocyanins, in elderberries during juicing.

Purging of the elderberry juice with nitrogen and/or addition of ascorbic acid reduced the oxidative degradation rate of the antioxidants. The presence of vitamin C protected the anthocyanins, but not quercetin from oxidative degradation. Mixing fruits with air during processing and even a low content of oxygen in the juice before bottling must be avoided to preserve antioxidant quality.

Improvement of the nutritional value of the elderberry or wolfberry juice, and increased protection of antioxidants against degradation, may potentially be obtained by selection of berry cultivars having a higher content of vitamin C.

20. Fuleki T, Ricardo-Da-Silva JM. Department of Plant Agriculture, University of Guelph, Vineland Station, Ontario, Canada. **Effects of cultivar and processing method on the contents of catechins and procyanidins in grape juice.** J Agric Food Chem. 2003 Jan 29;51(3):640-6.

This work studied the effect of pressing method, pasteurization, cultivar, and vintage on the content of catechin, epicatechin, and procyanidins in grape juice. The results showed that the concentration of these flavanols in the juice was influenced, in decreasing order of importance, by pressing method, cultivar, pasteurization, and vintage. Cold pressing without maceration was the least and hot pressing after maceration at 60 degrees C for 60 min the most effective method for extracting the flavanols. Pasteurization increased the concentration of catechins in cold-pressed juices, but it decreased concentrations in hot-pressed juices. The concentration of most procyanidins was increased by pasteurization.

21. Mazza G, Kay CD, Cottrell T, Holub BJ. Food Research Program, Pacific Agri-Food Research Centre, Agriculture and Agri-Food Canada, Summerland, British Columbia, Canada. **Absorption of anthocyanins from blueberries and serum antioxidant status in human subjects.** J Agric Food Chem. 2002 Dec 18;50(26):7731-7.

This research group examined the absorption from stomach to blood of anthocyanins after consumption of a high-fat meal (intended to promote absorption and bioavailability) with freeze-dried blueberry powder containing 25 individual anthocyanins. Nineteen of the blueberry anthocyanins were detected in human blood serum. Furthermore, the appearance of total anthocyanins in the serum was directly correlated with an increase in serum antioxidant capacity.

These results showed that anthocyanins are absorbed in their intact forms in humans and that consumption of blueberries, a food source with high antioxidant properties, is associated with a diet-induced increase in blood antioxidant status.

In a somewhat analogous study on wolfberry consumption, Yueng Chen and colleagues (reference below) fed human subjects 15 grams of whole wolfberries daily for 28 days. Blood zeaxanthin levels were studied and shown to be elevated on day 29, with increases 2.5x above the control subjects. This study demonstrated that blood zeaxanthin content could be increased by having wolfberries in the diet to blood levels significant for uptake of this carotenoid pigment into the retinal macula (see Chapter 5).

Reference for diet-induced increased in blood zeaxanthin content after eating wolfberries: Cheng CY, Chung WY, Szeto YT, Benzie IF. Antioxidant Research Group, Faculty of Health and Social Sciences, Hong Kong Polytechnic University, Hong Kong, China. **Fasting plasma zeaxanthin response to Fructus barbarum L. (wolfberry; Kei Tze) in a food-based human supplementation trial.** Br J Nutr. 2005 Jan;93(1):123-30.

22. Klopotek Y, Otto K, Bohm V., Institute of Nutrition, Friedrich Schiller University Jena, Jena, Germany, and Institute of Beverage Technology, University of Applied Sciences Lippe and Hoxter, Lemgo, Germany. **Processing strawberries to different products alters contents of vitamin C, total phenolics, total anthocyanins, and antioxidant capacity.** J Agric Food Chem. 2005 Jul 13;53(14):5640-6.

Strawberries were processed to juice, nectar, wine, and puree. For investigation of the antioxidant capacity as well as the contents of vitamin C (ascorbic acid), total phenolics and total anthocyanins, samples were taken after different stages of production to determine the effects of processing.

This study showed the decrease of all investigated parameters within processing strawberries to different products. *The content of vitamin C decreased with production time and processing steps, especially during heat treatment.* Fermentation did not lead to heavy losses of total phenolics. Total anthocyanins and the hydrophilic antioxidant capacity *decreased while using high temperatures.* Anthocyanins also decreased considerably during the processing of wines, mainly caused by fermentation and pasteurization.

23. Aaby K, Skrede G, Wrolstad RE, Matforsk AS, Norwegian Food Research Institute, Osloveien 1, N-1430 Aas, Norway. **Phenolic composition and antioxidant activities in flesh and achenes of strawberries (Fragaria ananassa).** J Agric Food Chem. 2005 May 18;53(10):4032-40.

In this study of strawberry pulp and achenes (single seeds), several phenolic acids and ORAC were determined for content changes during industrial processing. Phenolic acid levels and antioxidant activity of strawberry achenes were reduced by industrial processing. One major surprising result, however, was that the content of antioxidant phenolics was still high in the strawberry waste byproduct (sometimes called "presscake" or pomace), and thus could be a valuable source of nutraceuticals or natural antioxidants.

Summary:

Processing Variables Affecting Berry Nutrients

Although not intended to be comprehensive, this chapter helps reveal processing factors that can affect nutrient density and quality of wolfberries. Although much of the research has been done on other berries and common fruits, we infer the same effects would apply to wolfberry processing. We caution readers that these interpretations are speculative.

To summarize from the literature reviewed, there are at least 14 factors that manufacturers of wolfberry products may need to control, account for, or stipulate to fruit processors and consumers when reporting nutrient content of wolfberry raw materials

1. differences between species, cultivars, varietals
2. storage temperature
3. berry specie and fruit size
4. plant component(s) used for food or juice, especially retention of skin and seed where phytochemicals are localized
5. geography, climate, soil conditions of harvest
6. harvest time, ripening, and maturity characteristics
7. drying methods
8. type of solvent used for extractions
9. storage factors, such as use of oxygen, vitamin C, and exposure to light
10. cooking conditions such as intensity and duration of heat
11. maceration
12. juicing techniques, pressing methods, fermentation, pasteurization
13. phytochemical content of pomace after juicing
14. conditions affecting in vivo absorption, i.e., the bioavailability of digested wolfberry phytochemicals

As perhaps the most identifiable nutrient class in wolfberries, carotenoids particularly have attracted attention for their wide variety of applications in foods and their unusual value as dietary antioxidants.

As mentioned in Chapter 5's discussion of antioxidants, perhaps the ORAC measurement would be valuable on food labels, used as an index of nutrient quality and freshness after processing. It will be interesting to see over the coming years to what extent food labels report ORAC or some other representative parameter of antioxidant or nutrient preservation.

Below, we present an abstract of research specifically analyzing the *effects of processing on carotenoids*, providing a guide of factors likely important to retaining optimum levels of this nutrient class in processed wolfberries.

Publication. Rodriguez-Amaya DB. Food carotenoids: analysis, composition and alterations during storage and processing of foods. Departamento de Ciencia de Alimentos, Faculdade de Engenharia de Alimentos, Universidade Estadual de Campinas, Brasil. Forum Nutr. 2003;56:35-7.

Abstract. Substantial progress has been achieved in recent years in refining the analytical methods and evaluating the accuracy of carotenoid data. Although carotenoid analysis is inherently difficult and continues to be error prone, more complete and reliable data are now available. Rather than expressing the analytical results as retinol equivalents, there is a tendency to present the concentrations of individual carotenoids, particularly beta-carotene, beta-cryptoxanthin, alpha-carotene, lycopene, lutein and zeaxanthin, carotenoids found in the human plasma and considered to be important to human health in terms of the provitamin A activity and/or reduction of the risk for developing degenerative diseases.

With the considerable effort directed to carotenoid analysis, many food sources have now been analyzed in different countries. The carotenoid composition of foods varies qualitatively and quantitatively. Even in a given food, *compositional variability occurs because of factors such as stage of maturity, variety or cultivar, climate or season, part of the plant consumed, production practices, post-harvest handling, processing and storage of food.*

During processing, isomerization of trans-carotenoids, the usual configuration in nature, to the cis-forms occurs, with consequent alteration of carotenoid bioavailability and biological activity. Isomerization is promoted by light, heat and acids.

The principal cause of carotenoid loss during processing and storage of food is enzymatic or non-enzymatic oxidation of the highly unsaturated carotenoid molecules.

The occurrence and extent of oxidation depends on the presence of
- oxygen
- metals
- enzymes
- unsaturated lipids
- prooxidants, antioxidants
- exposure to light
- type and physical state of the carotenoids present

- severity and duration of processing
- packaging material
- storage conditions

Thus, retention of carotenoids is a major concern in the preparation, processing and storage of foods. [end of article]

As wolfberries gain popularity in western countries and become considered for a variety of functional food applications, it is likely that this fruit will undergo more intense regulatory scrutiny. Obtaining GRAS or GRAE status (in the USA, "Generally Regarded As Safe" and "Generally Regarded As Efficacious") will require better understanding of wolfberry's safety profile when taken in certain diets and therapeutic programs, pharmacological properties and interactions, bioavailability and toxicology under conditions of high intake for long durations.

In order to convince the food scientific community about wolfberry's health benefits and diversity of uses in functional foods and beverages, manufacturers of wolfberry products will have to consider a panel of science-based communications to provide confidence about the benefits of this berry.

Making leaps of faith and outlandish claims about improving health, "increasing sexual energy", adding years to life, curing cancer, etc. do not create credibility about the nutritional value of wolfberries or any food. Reasonable discussions will have to

- describe how wolfberries contribute to specific health advantages, overall health and a positive lifestyle, not as a single food but in a mixed diet
- convey in simple terms what the existing science is on wolfberry nutrients and how new science expands our understanding
- apply a degree of skepticism about potential health effects from long-term consumption of wolfberries until true effects are proven in clinical trials whose results are approved upon global standards
- for individual wolfberry nutrients or the whole fruit, state the food-value message as simply as possible in the context of available science
- where basic or clinical science has been applied relevant to a particular wolfberry health benefit, explain the specifics of study design, expert opinions, and overall body of evidence

- once wolfberry products are more common on western markets, give consumers reports of "in-market surveillance" to assure efficacy on dietary applications of wolfberry products

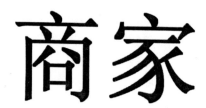

Where to Buy Dried Wolfberries or Other Wolfberry Raw Materials and Manufactured Products

If you cannot find wolfberry or goji berry products at a health food store close to you, they are available through mail order, direct sales, and the internet. The following companies provide good information on the origin, processing and quality control of imported wolfberries from China, as well as offering quality wolfberry products.

Rich Nature Nutraceutical Laboratories
http://www.richnature.com/
9700 Harbour Place, Suite 128
Mukilteo, WA 98275 USA
1-888-708-8127

Dried wolfberries, wolfberry concentrated pulp powder, wolfberry juice concentrate, wolfberry juice powder, wolfberry soap. An importer of wolfberry raw materials from Ningxia, Rich Nature provides wholesale, mail order and retail sales over its website. Rich Nature has collaborations with government and university laboratories by donating wolfberry raw materials for research and invites further proposals for scientific or horticultural studies of wolfberries. Contact Richard Zhang.

Young Living Essential Oils
http://www.youngliving.us/
Thanksgiving Point Business Park
3125 Executive Parkway
Lehi, UT 84043 USA
1-800-371-2928

Dried wolfberries, wolfberry puree juice ("NingXia Red"), wolfberry granola bar. Wolfberries from Ningxia. Young Living is a direct sales company.

Superfoods
http://www.livesuperfoods.com/
PO Box 524
Fall City, WA 98024 USA
1-800-481-5074

Dried wolfberries, concentrated wolfberry pulp powder. Wolfberries from Ningxia. Superfoods is a wholesale and mail order company.

FreeLife International
http://www.freelife.com/
333 Quarry Road
Milford, CT 06460 USA
1-800-882-7240

Wolfberry juice ("Himalayan Goji Juice"). Promotional literature says wolfberries are from Tibet. FreeLife is a direct sales company.

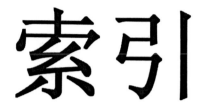

CHAPTER 11
Glossary of Terms, Index

A

Acai—*Euterpe oleracea*, Brazilian palmberry, thought by some to be Nature's most nutritious berry. Compared with wolfberry in Chapter 3.

Acetic acid, acetate—a short-chain fatty acid; produced by intestinal fermentation of polysaccharides, Chapter 4

Adjuvant—in medicine, an adjuvant modifies the effect of other agents while having few if any direct effects alone; Chapter 6

Agar—a tasteless extract from seaweed used for thickening foods or as a laboratory gel; Chapter 4.

Age-related macular degeneration, AMD—from ophthalmology, the progressive decline during aging of vision associated with defects in the retinal macula; Chapter 5

Alanine—an amino acid found in wolfberry, Chapter 3

Algae—photosynthetic aquatic plants including seaweeds that range in size from microscopic single cell forms to giant forms several meters long (kelp); origin of the carotenoid, astaxanthin, Chapter 4

Alpha-carotene—a carotenoid terpene found in wolfberries. It serves as a photosynthetic pigment and has antioxidant properties, Chapter 5

Alpha-galactosidase—deficiency of this enzyme leads to Fabry disease, a genetic disorder resulting from incomplete metabolism of essential lipids called glycosphingolipids. Wolfberry calystegines were shown to benefit patients with Fabry's disease, Chapter 6

Alpha-linolenic acid—a plant-based omega-3 fatty acid essential for good nutrition; found in wolfberry seeds, Chapter 3

Aluminum—a trace mineral present in wolfberries, Chapter 3

Amino acids—a class of 20 molecules that make up proteins in living organisms; all are present in wolfberries, Chapter 3

Anthocyanidin—a major subgroup of flavonoids found in all vascular plants. Forms the chemical structural backbone for anthocyanins. Suspected but not yet demonstrated in wolfberries. Described as "biological response modifiers", acting mainly as antioxidants, Chapters 3,5,10

Anthocyanin—(etymology: Greek. anthos = flower, kyáneos = purple) is a water soluble pigment that reflects the red to blue range of the visible spectrum. Often observed in plants where it serves to color fruits, leaves, bark, etc. The pigment acts as a powerful antioxidant helping to protect the plant from ultraviolet damage. Suspected to exist in wolfberries but not yet demonstrated, Chapters 3,5,10

Anti-aging—nutrients that may reduce, prevent, or reverse the decline of physiological function with increasing years, as attributed to consumption of wolfberries in Chinese legend. No valid proof exists for such an effect, Chapter 6

Antibacterial—a substance that destroys bacteria, or suppresses their growth or reproduction, properties that may be provided by wolfberries, Chapter 6

Antioxidant—certain vitamins and other nutrients that may provide protection from the damage caused by "free radicals" created as a result of oxygen reactions in living tissues. Wolfberry carotenoids provide antioxidant functions, Chapter 5

Antiviral—an agent that inhibits growth or multiplication of viruses, or kills them. Such properties may be provided by wolfberries, Chapter 6

Apigenin—plant flavonoid with antioxidant, anti-inflammatory and chemopreventive properties. Commonly found in apples, tomatoes, grapes, cherries and many other fruits and vegetables. May be present in wolfberries, Chapter 6

Apoptosis—genetically-fixed cell death occurring naturally as part of normal development, maintenance, or renewal of living plant and animal tissues. Wolfberries appear to stimulate apoptosis of cancer cells, Chapters 5,6

Arabinose—a simple sugar, resistant starch (dietary fiber) and carbohydrate source present in wolfberries, Chapter 3

AREDS—Age-Related Eye Disease Study, conducted by the US National Eye Institute, National Institutes of Health, showing that antioxidant nutrients—beta-carotene, vitamins A, C and E, and zinc, reduced progression of age-related macular degeneration in elderly patients; Chapters 5,6

Arginine—an amino acid involved in the Krebs cycle and a precursor of nitric oxide, the endothelium-derived relaxing factor important in control of capillary functions and blood pressure regulation; present in high concentration in wolfberries, Chapters 3,6

Arsenic—a naturally occurring element often used in pesticides and herbicides. Can accumulate to toxic levels, and is known to cause cancer in humans and other living things. Wolfberry polysaccharides may inhibit the effects of arsenic, Chapter 4

Arteries, arterioles—so-called "resistance" vessels of the vascular system important for maintenance of blood pressure and local blood flow in organs. Wolfberry-derived arginine may be an important dietary source for regulating these blood vessels; Chapters 3,6

Ascorbic acid (vitamin C)—a natural compound involved in collagen and bone formation having antioxidant properties. Found in high concentration in wolfberries, Chapter 3

Aspartic acid—an amino acid that promotes uptake of trace elements and is intricately involved with the energy cycle of the body; present in wolfberries, Chapter 3

Astaxanthin—a carotenoid pigment commonly found in marine species having yellow and red colors; not present in wolfberries, Chapter 5

Asteridae—botanical subclass of the plant family Solanaceae to which wolfberry belongs (Chapter 8); flowering plants in class Dicotyledon or Magnoliopsida. Like all other dicotyledons, their seed contains two embryonic leaves or cotyledons; Chapter 8

Astringent—a property of phenolics in edible plants having a sour, sometimes bitter taste. Considered to arise from phenolic tannins in species like cranberries and tea leaves; Chapter 10

B

Berry Young Juice—a multiple-ingredient juice made and marketed by Young Living Essential Oils. It contains wolfberry juice and the juices of several other fruits including blueberry, pomegranate, raspberry and apricot. Also contains lemon and orange essential oils, two strong antioxidant sources, Chapters 2,6

Betaine—(trimethylglycine) functions with choline, folic acid, vitamin B12, and methionine as "methyl donors," i.e., to carry and donate methyl molecules for chemical processes important to proper liver function, cellular replication, and detoxification reactions; present in wolfberries, Chapter 6

Beta-carotene—a tetraterpene, an orange photosynthetic pigment, important for plant photosynthesis and responsible for the red-orange hue of wolfberries and orange color of carrots; two forms—alpha and beta-carotene—both of which are stored in the liver; carotene is non-toxic and converted to vitamin A as needed; strong antioxidant properties, richly present in wolfberries, Chapters 3,5,6

Beta-cryptoxanthin—a carotenoid light-sensitive pigment having alpha and beta forms identical to alpha- and beta-carotene, respectively, except for an invariant cyclohexene ring; strong antioxidant properties, richly present in wolfberries, Chapters 3,5,6

Beta-glucan—a polysaccharide (long string of sugar molecules) obtained from oats and several types of mushrooms, a fermentable fiber, similar to wolfberry polysaccharides, Chapter 4

Beta-hydroxy beta-methylbutyrate (HMB)—a metabolite of the essential amino acid leucine, is a dietary supplement promoted to enhance gains in strength and lean body mass associated with resistance training; leucine levels are high in wolfberries, implicating a similar mechanism of benefit, Chapter 3

Beta-sitosterol—a plant steroid involved in fat metabolism, possibly with cholesterol-lowering and antioxidant properties, present in wolfberries, Chapter 3

Biotin—also known as vitamin B7 important in metabolism of fatty acids and the amino acid, leucine; may be present in wolfberries, Chapter 3

Black raspberries—Rubus occidentalis, a potent source of phenolic acid antioxidants, Chapter 10

Blood clotting—coagulation, a process possibly inhibited by wolfberry terpenes, Chapter 6

Blueberries—Vaccinium angustifolium (lowbush, wild) and corymbosum (highbush, cultivated), a potent source of phenolic antioxidants, Chapters 3,10

Botany and Botanical Taxonomy—the science concerned with the study, classification, structure, ecology and economic importance of plants; theory and practice of describing, naming and classifying plants, Chapter 8

Boxthorn—Lycium, a genus of about 100 species of plants in the Solanaceae family, native throughout most of the temperate zones of the world. Other names include Christmas berry, matrimony vine et al. shown in Chapter 8

Brix—an index of sweetness measured in fruit juice, established to estimate the ideal sugar content in grapes at the optimal time of harvesting (20-25); brix of wolfberry juice = 26, Chapter 3

Butyric acid, butyrate—a short-chain (4-carbon) saturated fatty acid beneficial to normal intestinal functions and mineral uptake; a product of fermentation such as from wolfberry polysaccharides, Chapter 4

C

Calcium—although approximately 99% of the body's calcium is contained in teeth and bone, calcium ions are required for muscle contraction, blood coagulation, enzyme activation, nerve impulse transmission, and changes in cell membrane and capillary permeability; high content present in wolfberries, Chapter 3

Calorie—common unit of energy equal to a kilocalorie (kcal) to describe amount of energy contained in food. One kcal raises the temperature of one kilogram of water by one degree Celsius; Chapter 3

Calystegine—an alkaloid (nitrogen-containing) typical of Solanaceous plants (as is wolfberry) that inhibits a large enzyme class called glycosidases having important roles in metabolism; Chapter 6

Cancer—uncontrolled cell division leading to growth of abnormal tissue that can invade and destroy healthy organs; believed that cancers arise from both genetic and environmental factors; may be beneficially affected by wolfberry nutrients, Chapters 4,5,6

Capillary—smallest blood vessel, located between an arteriole and a venule, whose thin wall permits diffusion of gases and nutrients between blood and organ fluids; Chapter 6

Carrageenan—a gel-forming polysaccharide found in red algae seaweed known as "Irish moss", used commercially in toothpastes and creamy processed foods; Chapters 4,6

Carbohydrate—one of the four main classes of macronutrients in food (also fats, fiber and proteins) and a source of energy; mainly sugars and starches that the body breaks down into glucose used as an energy source for cells; Chapter 3

Carcinogen—a substance capable of causing cancer; Chapters 4,6

Cardiovascular diseases—affect the heart and blood vessel system, such as coronary heart disease, heart attack, high blood pressure (hypertension), stroke, angina (chest pain); Chapter 6

Carotenoid—red, orange, purple or yellow plant pigments found in wolfberries; fat-soluble and widely used as food colorings; beta-carotene is precursor for formation of Vitamin A; particularly rich content in wolfberries, Chapters 3,5

Catalase—enzyme found in most plant and animal cells functioning to decompose hydrogen peroxide into hydrogen and water; Chapter 6

Cataract—a disorder of aging causing opacity or cloudiness of the eye's crystalline lens preventing a clear image from forming on the retina; Chapters 5,6

Catechin—a flavonoid with antioxidant properties, normally found in black and green teas; Chapter 10

Cellulose—a polysaccharide comprising the cell walls of plants; Chapters 4,6

Cerebroside—a lipid compound containing glucose or galactose found in the brain and other nervous tissue but having wide distribution also among plants; Chapters 3, 6

Chemotherapy—treatment with drugs to minimize the effects of cancer; Chapters 4,6

Christmas berry—a term given to wolfberry (Chapter 8) but usually applied to ornamental evergreen shrubs of the Pacific coast of the United States having large white flowers and red berrylike fruits; genus Photinia

Cholesterol—fat-like substance produced by the liver and found in the blood; present in food from fatty animal sources; Chapter 6

Clinical trial—carefully designed investigation of the effects of a medical treatment, including specific food extracts, on a group of human subjects; reference to wolfberry clinical trials, Chapters 3-5; general references Chapters 2-6,10

Colitis—inflammation of the large intestine, particularly the colon; Chapter 6

Colon—part of the large intestine between the cecum and the rectum; Chapter 6

Copper—a mineral and micronutrient serving as an internal catalyst and electron carrier; present in wolfberries, Chapter 3

Coumarin—extract from many plants including wolfberries (Chapter 6); has a sweet scent, readily recognized as the scent of newly-mown lawns and cut hay; has clinical value as precursor for anticoagulants, notably warfarin (coumadin); Chapter 6

Crohn's disease—chronic inflammatory disease of the digestive tract, typically the ileum; often associated with auto-immune disorders; Chapter 6

Cui Yueli—considered father of modern traditional Chinese medicine and former Chinese Minister of Health; Dedication and Chapter 7

Cultivar—cultivated variety of a plant selected for some feature that distinguishes it from the species from which it was selected; Chapter 8

Cystine—a naturally occurring amino acid; Chapter 3

Cytokines—low molecular weight proteins that stimulate or inhibit the proliferation or function of immune cells; Chapter 6

D

Daucosterol—sitosterol-D-glucoside and therefore likely the same as sitosterol; a steroidal alcohol, i.e., "phytosterol", possibly having antioxidant and cholesterol-lowering activities; found in wolfberries, Chapter 6

Diabetes—the condition in which the body does not produce or respond to insulin, a hormone produced in the pancreas promoting uptake of blood sugar (glucose) into body cells for energy; Chapters 4,6

Dicotyledons—flowering plants like wolfberry (Chapter 8) with two embryonic seed leaves or "cotyledons" appearing at germination

Dietary fiber—long-chain carbohydrates (polysaccharides) that are not digestible but are degraded by the human digestive tract into beneficial components sometimes grouped as "soluble" (in water) or "insoluble; soluble fibers are prebiotics providing food for intestinal bacteria; insoluble fibers are bulking agents aiding in laxation; wolfberry is a source of dietary fiber, particularly its polysaccharides, Chapters 3,4

Diverticulitis—inflammatory condition that occurs when small pouches in the colon (diverticula) become infected or irritated; Chapters 4,6

DNA—Deoxyribonucleic acid, a chemical found primarily in the cell nucleus; carries instructions for making all structures and materials the body needs to function, Chapter 4

Docosahexaenoic acid—DHA, an omega-3 fatty acid with 22 carbon atoms, the most unsaturated fatty acid available in the diet, high amounts of which are in fish and some plant oils, such as in flax seeds, Chapter 3

Duke of Argyll's tea plant—a name for wolfberry (Chapter 8) although common name is of 19th century origin refers to the 3rd Duke of Argyll who received this plant and a tea plant (*Camellia sinensis*) with their labels mixed up, and so grew it under the wrong label at his home in Middlesex, England

E

EDRF, endothelium-derived relaxing factor—nitric oxide synthesized from arginine; a dilating factor with multiple other roles in body physiology mainly as a short-acting signaling molecule between cells; rich in arginine, wolfberries may be a useful dietary source for EDRF formation, Chapter 6

Eicosapentaenoic acid—EPA, omega-3 fatty acid found in fish oils, marine plants and some plant oils, such as in flax seeds, Chapter 3; acts by producing eicosanoids which are involved in numerous physiological mechanisms, including inflammation control

Ellagic acid—phenolic antioxidant naturally found in plants in the form of ellagitannin; common in red, blue and black berries, reported as present in wolfberries, Chapter 3; although ellagic acid is the bioactive agent that offers antioxidant protection, the phytochemical is generally ingested in the naturally present ellagitannin form

Electrolyte—a substance in blood or body water that helps to regulate the overall balance of cell and body fluids; examples include sodium and potassium, both of which are richly contained in wolfberries, Chapter 3

EMEA, European Medicines Evaluation Agency—governs approval of medical products in the European Union, much like the FDA does in the US, Chapters 2,6,10

Endothelium, endothelial cells—the innermost layer of cells in blood vessels and the principal cell of capillaries, Chapter 6

Endothelium-derived relaxing factor—EDRF, nitric oxide, see EDRF above; Chapter 3.

Energy—output capability of a cell, battery, food consumed or work effort, usually expressed in watt-hours or calories expended, Chapter 3

Enzyme—a protein produced in the body to catalyze or facilitate a specific physiological response involving other substances without itself being destroyed or changed; wolfberry nutrients may be influenced by or induce enzymatic responses, Chapters 4-6

Enteritis—inflammation within the intestine; Chapters 4,6

Epicatechin—also includes epicatechin gallate, epigallocatechin, epigallocatechin gallate, a phenolic antioxidant found in green tea, Chapter 3,10

Epidemiology—study of the distribution and causes of disease occurrence in a population; Chapter 6

Epithelial cells—cells—some of which absorb nutrients—lining inner and outer surfaces of the body; Chapters 4,6

Epithet—in botany, the second name of the binomial for a plant, giving it specificity, e.g., "barbarum" is the specific epithet among genus Lycium to describe the wolfberry, Chapter 8

Erythrocytes—a synonym for oxygen-carrying red blood cells, Chapter 6

Essential nutrients—those nutrients that our bodies cannot make to meet demand of cell functions, e.g., some amino acids, vitamins, minerals and polyunsaturated fatty acids are essential, meaning that they must be consumed from the diet; Chapter 3

Extracellular fluid—all body fluids, including blood, other than the fluid within cells ("intracellular fluid"); Chapter 6

F

Fabry's disease—a fat storage disorder caused by a deficiency of an enzyme involved in the degradation of lipids; wolfberry calystegines may have beneficial effects, Chapter 6

Fat—found mainly in animal tissue and certain plants, including wolfberries (Chapter 3), a macronutrient that supplies calories to the body; there are 9 calories in each gram of fat—more than twice the calories in protein or carbohydrates

Fatty acid—long-chain molecule consisting of carbon, hydrogen and oxygen atoms that make up fat and essential oils in plants; omega-3 and omega-6 are plant fatty acids with health benefits and are present in wolfberries and flax seeds, Chapter 3

FDA, US Food and Drug Administration—US government agency whose mission is "to promote and protect the public health by helping safe and effective products reach the market in a timely way, and monitoring products for continued safety after they are in use"; includes review of plant extracts, Chapters 2,3,6

Feng shui—pronounced "fung shway" and meaning "wind-water", ancient Chinese art of incorporating and positioning objects to create balance and harmony through the flow of chi (energy), Chapter 7

Fermentation—occurring in the large intestine, energy-yielding metabolic breakdown of a nutrient molecule, such as a wolfberry polysaccharide, yielding short-chain fatty acids and a variety of other healthful nutrients and benefits, Chapter 4

Ferulic acid—a hydroxycinnamic acid and therefore a phenolic acid antioxidant possibly present within wolfberries, Chapter 6

Fiber—see, dietary fiber; Chapters 3,4

Fibrosis—development of excess fibrous connective tissue in an organ, Chapter 6

Flavonoid—a group of polyphenols including flavonols, flavones, flavanones, flavan-3-ols and anthocyanidins with antioxidant and anti-inflammatory properties; found in dark berries, seeds, roots, leaves, vegetables and cocoa; may be present in wolfberries, Chapters 3,6,10

Flora—a collective term for plant life, Chapter 8

Folic acid, folate—a B vitamin commonly obtained from green leafy vegetables like spinach; essential for synthesis of DNA and therefore growth and division of cells; may be present in wolfberries, Chapter 3

Fovea—central area of the eye's retina containing the densest concentration of photoreceptors (cones only) where the highest resolution visual processing is initiated; possibly supported by dietary carotenoids from wolfberry consumption, Chapters 3,5,6

Free radical—see radical oxygen specie; Chapter 5

Fructose—a fermentable 6-carbon monosaccharide or sugar found in fruits and honey; present in wolfberries, Chapters 3,4

Fructus lycii—a synonym for Lycium barbarum L., wolfberries, Chapter 8

Functional food—"consumed as part of a usual diet that is similar in appearance to, or may be, a conventional food, and is demonstrated to have physiological benefits and/or reduce the risk of chronic disease beyond basic nutritional functions." (Health Canada); Chapters 2-6,10

G

Galactose—a monosaccharide, a constituent of many oligo—and polysaccharides occurring in fruits as fermentable fiber such as gums, pectins and mucilages; present in wolfberries, Chapter 3

Gallic acid—a plant polyphenolic having antioxidant properties; may be present in wolfberries, Chapter 6

Ganoderma lucidum (Reishi mushroom)—also known as Ling zhi meaning "herb of spiritual potency". Ganoderma mushrooms have been used for more than 4000 years in Traditional Chinese Medicine; has abundant nutrients and polysaccharides that may be similar in structure and function to those of wolfberries, Chapter 4

Gansu—a province in north-central China where wolfberries have grown for thousands of years, region of Loess Plateau immediately west of Ningxia, Chapter 9

Genistein—a phenolic isoflavone antioxidant found in soy products; being studied for potential application as anti-cancer agents; Chapter 6

Germanium—a trace mineral found in wolfberries, Chapter 3

Glucose—a six-carbon fermentable monosaccharide formed from carbohydrate metabolism, a sugar used in plants and animals for energy; the main circulating energy source for cell functions; found in wolfberries, Chapter 3

Glutamic acid—a natural amino acid involved in protein synthesis; present in wolfberries, Chapter 3

Glycan—a type of polysaccharide sometimes bound to proteins, making a proteoglycan found in connective tissue; Chapter 6

Glycemic index—a numerical index given to a carbohydrate-rich food that is based on the average increase in blood glucose levels occurring after the food is eaten; wolfberry has a low glycemic index, Chapters 3,6

Glycine—a natural amino acid present in wolfberries; an inhibitory transmitter in the nervous system, Chapter 3

Glycoconjugate—a molecule with one or more sugars attached to a protein or a lipid; Chapter 6

Goji fruit—a wolfberry specie some claim grows in the Himalayan Mountains of Tibet although there are no scientific reports confirming this growing region; Chapter 8

Goji Juice—a wolfberry juice made and marketed by FreeLife International, containing organic black cherry juice concentrate, pear juice concentrate, apple juice concentrate as main ingredients, Chapters 2,6

Gou qi zi, gouji fruit—Chinese terms for wolfberry, Chapter 8

gou qi ye—Chinese term for wolfberry leaves, Chapter 8

GRAE, Generally Regarded As Efficacious—substances intentionally added to food that do not require a formal premarket review by the US FDA to assure their efficacy because their efficacy has been established by prior applications in foods; Chapter 10

GRAS, Generally Regarded As Safe—substances intentionally added to food that do not require a formal premarket review by the US FDA to assure their safety because their safety has been established by a long history of use in foods; Chapter 10

H

Health Canada—the federal department responsible for helping Canadians maintain and improve their health; provides national leadership to develop health policy, enforce health regulations, promote disease prevention and enhance healthy living for all Canadians; Over 50% of Canadians now consume natural health products in the form of traditional herbal products, vitamins and mineral supplements, and homeopathic preparations. To ensure that these products are safe, in 1999, Health Canada established the Natural Health Products Directorate; Chapters 2,3,6

Heart disease—any number of diseases related to the heart and blood vessels, the most prevalent of which is coronary artery disease. When grouped together, these diseases are the leading cause of death in the United States; Chapter 6

Hebei—meaning "north of the (Yellow) River", Hebei is a province in north-east China where wolfberries have grown for centuries, Chapter 9.

Hepatoprotection—protection of the liver, Chapter 6.

Herpes simplex—a common, contagious, incurable, and in some cases sexually transmitted disease caused by a virus; can also affect the brain, in which case the consequent disease is called herpes simplex encephalitis; Chapter 6.

Himalaya Mountains—a mountain range extending some 2000 km on the border between India and Tibet; this range contains Everest, the world's highest mountain; goji berries, a variant of wolfberries, are said to grow in the foothills of these mountains, Chapter 9.

Histidine—an essential amino acid found in proteins that is important for the growth and repair of tissue; present in wolfberries, Chapter 3.

HIV-AIDS—human immunodeficiency virus-acquired immune deficiency syndrome; AIDS is caused by HIV; Chapter 6.

Homeostasis—the physiological process by which internal systems of the body (e.g., blood pressure, body temperature, acid-base balance) are maintained at equilibrium despite variations in the external conditions; Chapter 6.

Hormone—a chemical messenger within the body secreted by one type of cell, traveling via the blood or extracellular fluid to act on another type of cell; Chapter 6.

HPLC—high-performance liquid chromatography, a type of column chromatography using a combination of techniques to separate individual nutrients at high resolution; example, wolfberry carotenoids have been isolated and quantified by HPLC, Chapter 5.

Huang He (Yellow River)—China's second longest river (after the Chang Jiang) whose banks and flood plains in central China regions such as Ningxia have produced the highest quality wolfberries for thousands of years, Chapter 9.

Hydrophilic—a substance that absorbs, dissolves in or is attracted to water; Chapters 2,3,6.

Hydroxybenzoic acid—an antimicrobial agent related to Parabens used as a food preservative; Chapters 6,10.

Hydroxycinnamic acid—a phenolic acid flavonoid with antioxidant properties found in several dark berries; possibly present in wolfberries, Chapters 6,10.

Hypertension—abnormally high blood pressure, Chapter 6.

Hypoxia—abnormally low oxygen content in organs and tissues of the body; Chapter 6.

I

Immune system—complex system in the body responsible for fighting disease. Its primary function is to identify foreign substances in the body (bacteria, viruses, fungi or parasites) and develop a defense against them. This defense is known as the immune response. It involves production of protein molecules called antibodies to eliminate foreign organisms that invade the body; Chapters 4,6.

Immunoactivity—ability of substances such as wolfberry polysaccharides to evoke immune responses, Chapters 4,6.

Insoluble (fiber)—not soluble in water, fiber such as from the bran layer of grains that increases the rate at which food passes through the digestive tract; cellulose, hemicellulose and lignin are three prevalent sources of insoluble fibers; Chapters 4,6

Insulin—a hormone from the pancreas secreted to stimulate the uptake of glucose by body cells; Chapter 6.

Interleukins—a group of cytokines made by white blood cells (leukocytes, hence the—leukin) affecting function of the immune system; Chapters 4,6.

Inulin—naturally occurring oligosaccharides (several simple sugars linked together) produced by many types of plants; belong to a class of soluble fermentable fibers known as fructans; Chapter 4.

In vitro—literally, "in glass"; in a laboratory dish or test tube; an artificial environment; Chapters 4-6

In vivo—literally, "in life"; in living organisms like experimental animals or humans; Chapters 4-6.

Iron—an essential mineral forming part of hemoglobin, the protein in blood that carries oxygen throughout the body; rich content in wolfberries, Chapter 3.

Isoflavonoid—a phenolic antioxidant present in dark berries, fruits and vegetables, Chapters 3,6.

Isoleucine—an essential amino acid found in wolfberries, Chapter 3.

J (no entries)

K

Kaempferol—a flavonoid antioxidant present in many fruits and vegetables, including wolfberries, Chapters 6,10

Kau kei chi—a Cantonese term for wolfberry, Chapter 8

Kei tze—a Chinese term for wolfberry, Chapter 8

Kugicha—a Korean term for wolfberry, Chapter 8

Kukoshi—a Japanese term for wolfberry, Chapter 8

L

LBP—Lycium barbarum polysaccharide, the designation given to some

8 polysaccharides isolated from wolfberries, all of which have potential health properties following intestinal fermentation, Chapters 4,6.

Leucine—an essential amino acid found in wolfberries, Chapter 3.

Leukocyte—white blood cell that defends the body against viruses and bacteria; wolfberry nutrients may stimulate leukocyte formation, Chapter 6.

Linoleic acid—an essential omega-6 fatty acid that serves as the parent compound in the synthesis of other omega-6 fatty acids such as arachidonic acid; wolfberry seeds are rich in content of linoleic acid, Chapter 3.

Linolenic acid—an essential omega-3 fatty acid from oily fish (salmon) and certain plants, such as flax (Chapter 3); may reduce the risk of cardiovascular disease and myocardial infarction by lowering triglyceride levels and blood pressure and preventing the formation of life-threatening blood clots

Linnaeus—Carl, Swedish botanist who devised the modern system of botanical nomenclature (1707-1778); Chapter 8.

Lipophilic—describes a substance that dissolves in or is attracted to fats, oils or other lipids. Lipophilic functional groups or molecules prefer to be in an environment where there is no water, such as wolfberry carotenoids, Chapter 5

Lutein—pronounced "loo-teen", a carotenoid pigment in the xanthophyll class, present in wolfberries and spinach (Chapters 3,5). Found in high concentrations in the retinal macula lutea of the posterior eye, and has been shown to protect against blindness caused by macular degeneration by light-filtering and antioxidant functions, Chapter 5

Luteolin—a citrus flavonoid antioxidant with anti-inflammatory and anti-tumor properties. Found in high amounts in parsley, thyme, and peppermint; may be present in wolfberries, Chapter 6

Lycium barbarum L.—the specie of wolfberry common to central and western China, Chapters 8,9.

Lycium chinense—a cultivar of Lycium barbarum L. found throughout China, Chapters 8,9.

Lycopene—a carotenoid with strong antioxidant properties found in tomatoes; not reported to exist in wolfberries, Chapters 3,6,10.

Lysine—an essential amino acid with roles in tissue repair and growth, found in wolfberries, Chapter 3.

M

Macronutrient—essential nutrients needed by the human body in large quantities (multiples of grams) for it to function normally. They include carbohydrates, proteins, fats, fiber and water—all provided in wolfberry fruit; Chapters 2,3,6.

Macula lutea—a yellowish central area of the retina rich in rods and cones as photoreceptors for perceiving light and images into clear detailed vision; pigmented yellow by dietary carotenoids, zeaxanthin and lutein, both rich in wolfberries, Chapters 3,5,6.

Macular degeneration—leading cause of blindness in individuals over age 60; two main types, dry and wet. The dry or atrophic type is the most common, affecting nearly 70 percent of all cases; results from macular tissues aging and breaking down, causing a gradual vision loss. May be prevented by increasing intake of dietary antioxidants, possibly by consuming wolfberries, Chapters 3,5

Magnesium—essential element influencing many enzymes needed to produce cellular energy and impulse transmissions in nerves and muscles; affecting general functions of the nervous, muscular and cardiovascular systems. Found mainly in bone and muscle; rich content in wolfberries, Chapter 3.

Magnoliophyta—flowering plants including wolfberry that produce seeds enclosed in an ovary, Chapter 8.

Magnoliopsida—flowering plants including wolfberry whose seed contains two embryonic leaves or cotyledons; Chapter 8.

Malondialdehyde (MDA)—a byproduct of lipid (fat) metabolism in the body also found in many foods; in diabetes, a biochemical marker of oxidative damage; its formation is possibly inhibited by wolfberry phytochemicals, Chapter 6.

Manganese—an essential trace mineral required in synthesis and regulation of enzymes involved in metabolism of proteins and fat. Supports immune functions, carbohydrate metabolism, production of cellular energy, reproduction and bone growth; rich content in wolfberries, Chapter 3.

Mannose—a 6 carbon sugar often a component of polysaccharides; present in wolfberries, Chapter 3.

Matrimony vine—any of various shrubs or vines of the genus Lycium with showy flowers and bright berries, including wolfberries, Chapter 8.

Metamucil—a popular dietary fiber supplement made from ground psyllium seed husks, Chapter 4.

Metastasis—in cancer, the migration of cancer cells from the original tumor site through blood, lymph or extracellular fluid to other tissues, Chapter 6.

Methionine—a sulfur containing amino acid, required for protein synthesis; present in wolfberries, Chapter 3.

Micronutrient—essential nutrient needed only in small quantities (milligrams or usually micrograms) to provide nutritional benefit; includes vitamins and minerals, as present in wolfberries, Chapter 3.

Mineral—an inorganic compound needed by the body for good health, proper metabolic functioning, and disease prevention. Examples are calcium, magnesium, and iron; more than 20 minerals present in wolfberries, Chapter 3

Molybdenum—a trace mineral with a role in enzyme systems involved in metabolism of carbohydrates, fats, and proteins; also found in tooth enamel; present in wolfberries, Chapter 3.

Monosaccharide—a sugar (like sucrose or fructose) that does not hydrolyze to give other sugars; the simplest group of carbohydrates; present in wolfberries, Chapters 3,4.

Monomenthyl succinate—an agent used experimentally to induce secretion of hormones from isolated preparations like islet or liver cells; interactions by wolfberry nutrients, Chapter 6.

Morali—Japanese name for wolfberry, Chapter 8.

Mucillage—the class of dietary fiber to which psyllium belongs, Chapters 3,4.

Mucin—lubricants composed of carbohydrate chains linked to proteins; structure and function possibly affected by wolfberry phytochemicals, Chapter 6.

Murali—Japanese term for wolfberry, Chapter 8.

Myricetin—a plant flavonoid with antioxidant properties, possibly contained in wolfberries, Chapter 3

N

Naringenin—a citrus flavonoid with antioxidant properties, Chapter 3

Natural health products—naturally occurring organic compounds (e.g., plants or their extracts such as wolfberries) found in nature imparting nutritional or anti-disease benefits, Chapters 2,3,6.

Natural Products Directorate of Health Canada—the regulating authority for sale of natural health products in Canada, Chapters 2,3.

Niacin—vitamin B3, present in wolfberries, Chapter 3.

Nightshade—a genus (Solanum) of annuals, perennials, sub-shrubs, shrubs and climbers with attractive fruit and flowers. Some such as wolfberries bear edible fruit or other parts, and include tomato, potato and eggplant, Chapter 8.

Ning xia gou qi—Chinese for wolfberries from Ningxia, Chapter 8.

Ningxia—The Chinese autonomous region in north-central China often called "The Home of the Wolfberry" famous for its premium wolfberry fruit, Chapter 9.

NingXia Red Juice—a wolfberry juice made and marketed by Young Living Essential Oils; the 2nd generation of Berry Young Juice. Contains wolfberry fruit puree and so has desirable nutrients from skin, seeds, pulp and stem of the wolfberry plant. Ingredients otherwise the same as Berry Young Juice, Chapters 2,6.

Nitric oxide—a short-lived gas with chemical formula NO having an important cell-cell signaling role in numerous human processes; the endothelium-derived relaxing factor, EDRF formed from arginine (rich in wolfberries) and nitric oxide synthase, Chapter 3

Nobel Prize—an international award given every year since 1901, recognizing achievements in literature, economics, major fields of science, and peace; the 1998 prize in physiology or medicine was awarded for the discovery of biological nitric oxide (above); Chapter 3.

O

Ocular—referring to the eyes and vision; potential benefit of wolfberry consumption, Chapters 3,5,6.

Oleic acid—an omega-9 unsaturated fatty acid found in various animal and vegetable sources, present in wolfberry seeds, Chapter 3.

Oligofructans—also called fructo-oligosaccharides, multiple chains of fructose sugar units providing an important source of fermentable dietary fiber, Chapter 4.

Omega fatty acids—a form of polyunsaturated fats, one of four basic types of fat that the body derives from food (cholesterol, saturated fat, and monounsaturated fat are the others.) All polyunsaturated fats, including the omega-3s (e.g., linolenic acid),—6s (e.g., linoleic acid) and—9s (e.g., oleic acid) are increasingly recognized as important to human health, Chapters 3,6.

Oncology—field of medicine devoted to the study of cancer and tumors encompassing all their characteristics—physical, chemical, genetic, biological, surgical, therapeutic, preventive; Chapter 6.

Oxidizing—taking place in the presence of oxygen, such as the damage caused to cellular constituents like DNA, proteins and lipids by reactive oxygen species (ROS, oxygen free radicals (below), Chapters 3,5,6.

Oxygen free radical—also called reactive oxygen specie (ROS), uncharged atomic or molecular specie with unpaired electrons or an otherwise open shell configuration. Highly reactive in body processes, so free radicals may take part in varied chemical reactions, some of them undesirable, Chapter 3,5

P

p-coumaric acid—an intermediate product of the phenylpropanoid pathway in plants, known to have potent antioxidant properties. Exists in wolfberries, Chapter 6.

pH—"potential" (of) "hydrogen" is a scientific measure of the activity of hydrogen ions in a solution and, therefore, its acidity or alkalinity; pH of soil may be an important determinant of nutrient density in wolfberries, Chapter 8.

p-hydroxybenzoic acid—an extract of wolfberries (Chapter 6) and a synonym for p-salicylic acid having anti-inflammatory, anti-pyretic (anti-fever) and anti-coagulant properties.

Palmitic acid—also called hexadecanoic acid, is one of the most common saturated fatty acids found in animals and plants, including wolfberry seeds, Chapter 3.

Pantothenic acid—also called vitamin B5, is an antioxidant water-soluble vitamin needed for the metabolism of carbohydrates, proteins, and fats. May be present in wolfberries, Chapter 3.

Papaya—Native to the Caribbean and North American sub-tropics, papaya is a large golden yellow fruit when ripe with an exotic sweet-tart flavor. Sometimes called pawpaw, some authors refer to it as one of the world's healthiest foods, Chapter 3.

Parasite—an animal or plant living in or on a host (another animal or plant); the parasite obtains nourishment from the host without benefiting or killing it. Wolfberry polysaccharides may have anti-parasitic activity, Chapters 4,6.

Pectin—present in wolfberries (Chapters 3,4), pectin is a polysaccharide (therefore, a dietary fiber) capable of producing a gel and hence has important setting properties, particularly, in the production of jams.

Phenolic acid, phenolics—also called phenols and polyphenols, this is a class of chemical compounds that include pigments and tannins with strong antioxidant activities and varied putative health benefits. Found in dark berries mainly in skin, seeds and stems. May be present in wolfberries, Chapters 3,6.

Phenolic amide—a caffeoyltyramine with strong antioxidant activity found in the root bark of wolfberries, Chapter 6.

Phenylalanine—an essential amino acid found in wolfberries (Chapter 3); a component of proteins and needed for growth of children and for protein metabolism in children and adults; normally converted to tyrosine in the human body

Phosphorus—an essential mineral found in nature combined with oxygen as phosphate; most phosphate in humans is in bone. Phosphate-containing molecules (phospholipids) are also important components of cell membranes and lipoproteins. Found in high concentration in wolfberries, Chapter 3.

Photo-oxidative damage—when light energy absorbed by plants becomes excessive relative to the capacity of photosynthesis, oxidation effects may include disruption of membranes. Also occurs in the human retina exposed to intense blue light. Wolfberry carotenoids may protect against these effects, Chapters 3,5,6.

Phytochemical—any chemical or nutrient derived from a plant source, see Chapters 2,3; may not be essential for normal functioning of any cell or organ but which nonetheless has beneficial effects for overall health; example, antioxidant pigments

Phytoestrogen—a naturally occurring compound of wolfberries (Chapters 3,6), that acts like estrogen in the body

Phytonutrient—a phytochemical with proven or suspected health promoting properties. Wolfberry vitamins and carotenoids are examples of phytonutrients, Chapters 2-6.

Pigment—any plant or animal cell material resulting in color from selective absorption. In wolfberries, the carotenoids are pigments for the fruit's orange-red color, Chapters 3,5.

Pigment power—a term used in lay publications referring to the antioxidant qualities and health benefits of berries, fruits and vegetables with bright colors, Chapter 5.

Plantae (kingdom of plants)—taxonomic kingdom consisting of vegetable organisms having chlorophyll that enables them to make food from photosynthesis, Chapter 8.

Plantago ovata—psyllium, a plant also known as "fleawort," valued for its high fiber content. The powdered seeds of this plant are often used as a laxative such as in Metamucil; Chapters 3,4.

Polyfructose, oligofructose—a sugar or carbohydrate soluble fiber source also known as fructopolysaccharide; the hydrolysis product of inulin and consists of 3 to 5 sugar units comprised of fructose and a terminal glucose. May be present in wolfberries, Chapters 3,4,6.

Polyp—a smooth-coated abnormal growth (tumor) projecting from a mucous membrane such as the intestine or colon; wolfberry polysaccharides may reduce polyp formation in the intestinal system, Chapters 4,6.

Polymerase—a class of enzymes that catalyze the formation of new DNA and RNA from an existing strand of DNA or RNA; stimulated by wolfberries, Chapter 6.

Polyphenol—see above, Phenolics

Polysaccharide—a carbohydrate source of dietary fiber consisting of a long chain—perhaps tens of thousands—of simple sugar molecules linked together. Starch and cellulose are examples. Fermentation yields numerous healthful byproducts, such as short-chain fatty acids; prevalent literature on Ganoderma mushrooms and wolfberries indicates polysaccharides may have profound health benefits, Chapter 4.

Polyunsaturated fat—a fatty acid with more than one double bond (C=C) in the carbon chain. Linoleic acid, having a rich content in wolfberries, is an example, Chapter 3.

Pomegranate—*Punica granatum L.*, a species of fruit-bearing deciduous shrub or small tree native from the mid-East to India; large globular fruit having many seeds with juicy red pulp reported with high nutrient density and strong antioxidant activity resulting from a high content of phenolics, Chapters 3,6.

Potassium—an essential element found primarily in cells where it has roles in membrane, muscle and nerve function and in metabolic processes. High concentration in wolfberries, Chapter 3.

Powerfood—a lay term for nutrient richness in a particular food source such as wolfberry, Chapter 3.

Prebiotic—a natural or synthetic substance that supports or nurtures growth of probiotics like bacteria. Most dietary prebiotics are poly— or oligosaccharides not digested in the upper gastrointestinal system but when in the colon provide a source of nutrition for probiotics—the beneficial bacteria. Wolfberry polysaccharides are prebiotics, Chapter 4.

Probiotic—bacterial cultures intended to assist the body's naturally occurring flora within the digestive tract. Many probiotics are present in natural sources such as lactobacillus of yogurt, Chapter 4.

Proline—an amino acid found in many proteins, especially collagen. Present in wolfberries, Chapter 3.

Propionic acid, propionate—a naturally occurring carboxylic acid, one of the short-chain fatty acids formed from metabolism of fermentable fibers in the colon. Wolfberry polysaccharides are likely a significant source, Chapter 4.

Prostaglandins—a group of fatty acid compounds with numerous effects throughout the body, including activity in inflammation, smooth muscle contraction, regulating body temperature, and effects on certain hormones; wolfberry nutrients may interact with prostaglandins, Chapter 6.

Protein—a molecule composed of amino acids linked together in a particular order specified by a gene's DNA sequence. Perform a wide variety of functions in the cell, including as enzymes, structural components, or signaling molecules. Wolfberry protein content, Chapter 3.

Protocatechuic acid—a phenolic antioxidant that may be present in wolfberries, Chapter 6.

Provitamin—a substance that is converted into a vitamin in animal tissues, e.g., beta-carotene, rich in wolfberries, is a provitamin for vitamin A, Chapter 3.

Psyllium—see *Plantago ovata L.*, above

Pyridoxine, vitamin B6—essential for metabolism of amino acids and starch molecules; may be present in wolfberries, Chapter 3.

Pyrrole—an organic compound contained in chlorophyll of plants and vitamin B12; may be present in wolfberries, Chapters 3,6.

PubMed—the online database of medical literature citations compiled by the US National Center for Biotechnology Information, National

Library of Medicine, National Institutes of Health, Bethesda, MD; Chapters 3-6,10.

Q

Qi—also "chi", the circulating life energy that in Chinese philosophy is thought to be inherent in all things; in traditional Chinese medicine the balance of negative and positive qi in the body is believed to be essential for good health; Chapter 7

Qinghai—a Chinese province named after the enormous Qinghai Lake (Koko Nor); Chapter 9

Quench—to extinguish or absorb completely, as antioxidant chemicals do to radical oxygen species; Chapters 3,5,6

Quercetin—a flavonol of the flavonoid family of phenolic antioxidants, commonly found in blue, black or red berries and attributed with a variety of health benefits; not known to exist in wolfberries, Chapters 3,6,10

R

Radical oxygen specie, ROS—reactive oxygen-containing free radicals generated during oxidative metabolism. ROS can react with and damage lipids, proteins, and DNA in cells, causing oxidative stress. Include hydrogen peroxide, superoxide radicals, and hydroxyl radicals; wolfberry antioxidant nutrients may inhibit ROS, Chapters 3,5,6

RDI—Recommended Dietary Intake, estimates of daily minimal dietary intake of established nutrients provided by the US National Academy of Sciences and Health Canada; see Chapter 3

Reishi mushroom—*Ganoderma lucidum*, mushroom known in China as Lingzhi; well studied for its phytochemicals and a variety of possible health properties, Chapter 4

Retina—light-sensitive tissue at the back of the eye containing rods and cones as photoreceptors that transmit light and visual images via the optic nerve to the brain. Its macula lutea is rich in zeaxanthin and lutein found in wolfberries, Chapters 3,5,6

Retinol—the dietary form of vitamin A; a fat-soluble, antioxidant vitamin important in vision and bone growth belonging to the family of retinoids. Retinol is ingested in a precursor form from plants (wolfberries, carrots, spinach) containing carotenes, Chapters 3,5,6.

Rhamnitol—a naturally occurring sugar alcohol found in wolfberries, likely adding to the brix (sweetness) value of wolfberries and having roles in calcium absorption and bone metabolism, Chapter 3

Rhodopsin—also known as visual purple, it is a photoreceptor protein located in the retinal rods and formed in the dark. When light strikes, the rhodopsin molecule changes shape, generating the initial signal in visual interpretation. Wolfberry consumption may increase rhodopsin concentration, Chapters 3,5,6.

Ribes—pronounced "r-eye-bees", the genus of flowering plants that yield berries called currants, black and red, Chapter 10

Riboflavin—also known as vitamin B2, an easily absorbed, water-soluble micronutrient with a key role in general metabolism of fats, carbohydrates, and proteins. It is essential for healthy skin, nails, hair growth and general good health; rich content in wolfberries, Table 4, Chapter 3.

ROS, radical oxygen species—see above, radical oxygen specie

RNA—ribonucleic acid involved in synthesis of proteins, Chapter 6.

Rubus—pronounced "roo-bus", a genus of berry plants in the family Rosaceae, subfamily Rosoideae, growing on brambles with fruit such as the blackberry, raspberry and boysenberry, "caneberries", Chapter 10.

S

Saturated fat—a form of fat in meat, coconut and palm oils, and animal sources such as whole-milk and dairy products; becomes firm at room temperature. These fats raise blood cholesterol levels, particularly LDL ("bad" cholesterol) levels; Chapter 3.

Scavenger—in describing antioxidant effects, a scavenger is a chemical agent counteracting the effects of impurities; wolfberry nutrients are probably scavengers of radical oxygen species, Chapters 3,5,6.

Scopoletin—a dietary coumarin possibly having roles in regulating blood pressure and anti-bacterial and anti-inflammatory actions; found in wolfberries, Chapter 6.

Seabuckthorn—*Hippophae rhamnoides L.*, a berry vine native to China having a rich nutritional profile, Chapter 10

Selenium—an essential trace mineral as a cofactor for glutathione peroxidase, an enzyme involved in the neutralization of free radicals; rich content in wolfberries, Chapters 3,6.

Serine—a common amino acid involved in cysteine formation; present in wolfberries, Chapter 3.

Shanxi—a northern province of China where wolfberries grow, Chapter 8.

Shen Nung—also Sheng Nung, pronounced "Shay-nun", from Chinese legend, the "Divine Healer" and father of Chinese agriculture, supposed discoverer of tea making from leaves, circa 2800 BC, Chapter 7

Short-chain fatty acids—formed from bacterial degradation of fermentable fibers such as wolfberry polysaccharides in the large intestine, contributing numerous byproducts (short-chain fatty acids) with potential health benefits, Chapter 4.

Silibinin—a phenolic flavonoid extract from milk thistle, related to silymarin, and present in wolfberries, having anti-proliferative and apoptosis-stimulating properties on cancer cells in vitro, Chapter 6.

Silybin—extracted from the seeds of Silybum marianum and possibly from wolfberries, having antioxidant properties, Chapter 6.

Silymarin—see silibinin

Sinapic acid—a component of plant leaf cell walls, affecting structural firmness and utility as a food; possibly present in wolfberry leaves, Chapter 6.

Sodium—a mineral and essential nutrient helping to maintain blood volume, regulate body water balance and nerve membrane function; present in wolfberries, Chapter 3.

Solanaceae—pronounced "sol-an-ace-ee-eye", wolfberry's botanical family, a large and economically important group of herbs, shrubs, flowers and trees, including tomatoes, potatoes, tobacco and petunia, Chapter 8.

Solanales—the botanical order to which the Solanaceae family belongs (above), so includes wolfberries, Chapter 8.

Solanum—a large genus of plants in the family Solanaceae (above). including several nightshades and many poisonous or medicinal species like wolfberry, Chapter 8.

Soluble (fiber)—dietary fiber having an affinity for water, either dissolving or swelling to form a gel; it includes gums, pectins, mucilages, and hemicelluloses, and occurs in wolfberry (polysaccharides), fruits, vegetables, oats, barley, legumes, etc. Acts to decrease the rate of stomach emptying and increase food bulk transit time, binds bile acids increasing their excretion; Chapters 3,4,6.

Spermatophyta—the taxonomic division that includes all seed-bearing plants, including wolfberries, Chapter 8.

Stearic acid—a natural fatty acid common in animal and vegetable fat sources, including wolfberry seeds. An emulsifying agent used in skin creams, deodorants, and lotions; Chapter 3.

Sterol—a subgroup of steroids that are lipids including cholesterol, phytosterols, and some steroid hormones; Chapter 3

Stroke, ischemic—temporary or permanent loss of blood supply to the brain, possibly minimized by blueberry consumption (via phenolic antioxidants), Chapter 6.

Strontium—a naturally occurring trace element found in wolfberries, Chapter 3.

Sucrose—a 2-unit sugar or diglyceride composed of glucose and fructose, present in wolfberries, Chapter 3.

Superfood—a lay term popularized in the book, *SuperFoods Rx* by Pratt and Matthews (references for Chapter 2), represents a high-nutrient food source, Chapters 2,3.

Superoxide dismutase, SOD—an enzyme that catalyzes conversion of the damaging radical oxygen specie, superoxide, into hydrogen peroxide and oxygen, neutralizing superoxide's activity; Chapter 6.

Synergy—two or more discrete dietary nutrients acting in concert to create a health effect greater than each has independently; Chapter 2,3.

Syringic acid—an antioxidant phenolic acid possibly present in wolfberries, Chapter 6.

T

Taosim—one of the great philosophical traditions in China, according to which an individual finds peace through quietly following the Tao, the "way"; Chapter 7

Taurine—non-essential amino acid that may be essential for development and maintenance of the central nervous system. Important for fat metabolism and blood cholesterol control; Chapter 6.

Taxonomy—biological discipline for classifying living organisms into groups based on shared characteristics; Chapter 8.

Terpenes, tri-terpenes—volatile organic hydrocarbons derived from the essential oil component of plants, possibly having health benefits. Found in Ganoderma mushrooms and wolfberries, Chapters 4-6.

Thiamin—vitamin B1, essential in metabolism helping cells to convert carbohydrates into energy; present in wolfberries, Chapter 3.

Threonine—essential amino acid needed for proper growth in infants and maintenance of nitrogen balance in adults; present in wolfberries, Chapter 3.

Thromboxane—an eicosanoid that increases stickiness of platelets and so contributes to blood clotting; may be inhibited by wolfberry polysaccharides, Chapter 6

Tocopherol—the antioxidant vitamin E, protecting cell membranes from oxidative damage; present in wolfberry leaves, Chapter 6.

Trace mineral—element present in minute but detectable quantities needed by the human body in small quantities usually at the microgram level; present in wolfberries, Chapter 3.

Tracheobionta—vascular plants having specialized cells that conduct water or sap within their tissues, including flowering plants such as the wolfberry; Chapter 8.

Traditional Chinese Medicine (TCM)—a sophisticated set of techniques, including acupuncture, herbal medicine, fung shui, food choices, acupressure, qi gong, and oriental massage applied to preventive practices and healing; emphasis on using natural food as a preventative, Chapter 7.

Tryptophan—an amino acid that occurs in proteins, is essential for growth and normal metabolism, and is a precursor of niacin and serotonin; present in wolfberries, Chapter 3.

Tumor-necrosis factor, TNF—a protein in the family of cytokines that function to destroy tumor cells and/or healthy cells; TNF may mediate disease progression in arthritis and cancer; may be inhibited by wolfberry polysaccharides, Chapter 4.

Tumor-suppressor gene—functions normally to stop cell growth, including inside cancerous tumors; wolfberries may stimulate these genes, Chapter 6.

Tyrosine—an amino acid found in most proteins; a precursor of several hormones, including dopamine, epinephrine, melatonin and thyroxine; present in wolfberries, Chapter 3.

U

USDA—United States Department of Agriculture, a Federal agency involved in all phases of agriculture. Oversees many regulations, agencies, pricing issues and grant opportunities; publisher of dietary guidelines for nutrient intake; Chapters 2,3,6,10

V

Vaccinium—a genus of berry shrubs in the plant family Ericaceae including the cranberry, blueberry, lingonberry, bilberry, and huckleberry. About 450 species found mostly in cool regions of the Northern Hemisphere; Chapters 3,10.

Valeric acid, valerate—a short-chain fatty acid formed from degradation of fermentable fibers in the large intestine; wolfberry polysaccharides are likely an important fiber source, Chapter 4.

Valine—an essential amino acid found in proteins; important for growth in children and nitrogen balance in adults; present in wolfberries, Chapter 3.

Vanadium—found naturally in many plants, a trace mineral that may help balance blood sugar levels; present in wolfberries, Chapter 3.

Vanillic acid—a methoxybenzoic acid (phenolic) that may be a pheromone and antioxidant; present in wolfberries, Chapter 6.

Varietal—usually applied to grape species for types of wines, term applies to a specific species variety of a plant as opposed to geographic or other designation; Chapters 8,9,10.

Vascular smooth muscle—type of smooth muscle found within and comprising the inner wall of blood vessels contributing to regulation of arterial blood pressure; Chapter 6.

Veins, venules—blood vessels that carry oxygen-poor blood from the capillary system back to the lungs and heart; Chapter 6.

Vitamin—an organic substance that acts as a cofactor and/or regulator of metabolic processes. There are 13 known vitamins, most of which are present in foods or supplements; some are produced within the body. Present in wolfberries, Chapter 3.

Vitamin A—retinol, a fat-soluble vitamin with multiple functions in the body, formed from the pro-vitamin A carotenoids, beta-carotene and beta-cryptoxanthin, rich in wolfberries, Chapters 3,5.

Vitamin B1—thiamin, a water-soluble nutrient necessary for the metabolism of fats and carbohydrates; present in wolfberries, Chapter 3.

Vitamin B2—riboflavin, an easily absorbed, water-soluble nutrient with a key role in maintaining human health supporting energy production and the metabolism of fats, carbohydrates, and proteins; present in wolfberries, Chapter 3.

Vitamin B3—niacin, nicotinaminde or nicotinic acid, a water-soluble vitamin having essential roles in energy metabolism; present in wolfberries, Chapter 3.

Vitamin B6—pyridoxine, a water-soluble vitamin essential for metabolism of amino acids and starch; may be present in wolfberries, Chapter 3.

Vitamin B12—cyanocobalamin or cobalamin, a water-soluble vitamin necessary for normal metabolism of nerve tissues and is active in carbohydrate, fat, and protein metabolism; may be present in wolfberries, Chapter 3.

Vitamin C—ascorbic acid, an essential water-soluble vitamin with many roles in human physiology, rich content in wolfberries, Chapters 3,10.

Vitamin E—tocopherol, a fat-soluble vitamin essential for normal reproduction and antioxidant functions that neutralize radical oxygen species; present in wolfberry leaves, Chapter 3.

Vitamin K—a fat-soluble vitamin, occurring in leafy green vegetables, tomatoes, and egg yolks, that promotes blood clotting and prevents hemorrhaging. Exists in several related forms; unknown if it exists in wolfberries, Chapter 3.

W

Warfarin—a commonly used anticoagulant, also known as Coumadin; possibly acts synergistically with wolfberry phytochemicals, Chapter 6.

Wolfberry—*Lycium barbarum L.*

X

Xanthophylls—yellow carotenoid pigments including *oxygenated* carotenoids such as lutein, beta-cryptoxanthin and zeaxanthin found in wolfberries, Chapter 5.

Xinjiang—the most northwestern autonomous region in China where wolfberries have grown for thousands of years, Chapter 9.

Xylose—a 5 carbon sugar found in wolfberries, Chapter 3.

Y

Yellow River—Huang He, a major river of north-central China where wolfberries have grown for centuries along its banks in yellow silt deposited by floods; flows west to east 5,463 km, the second longest river in China surpassed only by the Chang Jiang; Chapter 9

Yin/yang—concept originates in ancient Chinese philosophy describing two primal opposing but complementary forces found in all things in the universe; Chapter 7

Yinchuan—capital city of Ningxia Autonomous Region, China; Chapter 9

Z

Zeaxanthin dipalmitate—pronounced "zee-a-zan-thin", yellow carotenoid pigment extraordinarily rich in wolfberries, Chapters 3,5,6

Zinc—an essential mineral involved in protein synthesis, collagen formation and as a cofactor for more than 90 enzymes catalyzing antioxidant, immune and wound-healing functions; particularly rich content in wolfberries, Chapter 3

Zirconium—a trace metal found in wolfberries, Chapter 3

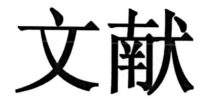

CHAPTER 12
References By Chapter, Useful Websites

Chapter 1—Introduction: Is Wolfberry Nature's Most Nutritious Food?

America's Obesity Crisis, Time Magazine Online, 2004
http://www.time.com/time/covers/1101040607/

Eat, Drink, and Be Healthy: The Harvard Medical School Guide to Healthy Eating, WC Willett, PJ Skerrett, 2002, Free Press, ISBN 0743223225

Food Fight: The Inside Story of the Food Industry, America's Obesity Crisis, and What We Can Do About It, KD Brownell, KB Horgen, McGraw-Hill, 2004, ISBN 0071438726

Functional Foods: Opportunities and Challenges, Institute of Food Technologists Expert Report, 2005

Gateway, total information resources of the US National Library of Medicine http://gateway.nlm.nih.gov

The Fat of the Land: Our Health Crisis and How Overweight Americans Can Help Themselves, M Fumento, Penguin Books, 1998, ISBN 0140261443

Chapter 2—Wolfberry Phytochemicals

Antioxidants and Cancer Prevention, US National Cancer Institute http://www.cancer.gov/newscenter/pressreleases/antioxidants

Berry Young Juice
http://berryyoungjuice.com

Clinical Trials for Natural Health Products, Natural Health Products Directorate, Health Canada
http://www.hc-sc.gc.ca/dhp-mps/prodnatur/legislation/docs/clini_trials-essais_nhp-psn_e.html

ClinicalTrials.gov, US National Institutes of Health
http://clinicaltrials.gov/

Dietary Guidelines for Americans, US Food and Drug Administration,
http://www.health.gov/dietaryguidelines/dga2000/document/frontcover.htm

Food and Nutrition Information Center, National Agriculture Library, US Department of Agriculture
http://www.nal.usda.gov/fnic/etext/000105.html

Functional Foods and Nutraceuticals: Biochemical and Processing Aspects, Vol. II, J Shi, G Mazza, M Le Mageur (Eds.), 2002, CRC Press, ISBN 1566769027

Goji Juice
http://gojiexpress.com/

Goji: The Himalayan Health Secret, E Mindell, R Handel, Momentum Media Health Series, 2003, ISBN 0967285526

NingXia Red Juice
http://ningxiared.com

Northwest Center for Small Fruits Research
http://www.nwsmallfruits.org/

Nutrient Database for Standard Reference, Agricultural Research Service, US Department of Agriculture
http://www.nal.usda.gov/fnic/foodcomp/search/

Office of Dietary Supplements, US National Institutes of Health http://ods.od.nih.gov/index.aspx

Oregon Berries
http://www.oregon-berries.com

Oregon State University College of Agricultural Sciences, Corvallis, http://agsci.oregonstate.edu/research/
Pacific Agri-Food Research Center, Agriculture and Agri-Food Canada, Summerland, British Columbia
http://res2.agr.ca/parc-crapac/summerland/progs/index_e.htm

Position Statement on Phytochemicals and Functional Foods, American Dietetic Association 1995
http://www.eatright.org/cps/rde/xchg/ada/hs.xsl/advocacy_adap1099_ENU_HTML.htm

PubMed, online database of health science publications from the US National Institutes of Health, National Center for Biotechnology Information, National Library of Medicine http://pubmed.gov/

Sea Buckthorn (Hippophae rhamnoides L.): production and utilization, TSC Li and THJ Beveridge, National Research Council of Canada Press, 2003, ISBN 0660190079, http://pubs.nrc-cnrc.gc.ca/cgi-bin/rp/rp2_book_e?mlist1_554

SuperFoods Rx, SG Pratt, K Matthews, HarperCollins Publishers, 2004, ISBN 0060535679

The Berry Bible, J Hibler, Morrow Cookbooks, 2004, ISBN 0060085487

The Superior Ningxia Wolfberry: A Powerful, Natural Ally Against Disease and Aging, H Rodier, MediaVision, 2005

US Department of Agriculture, Agricultural Research Services, Horticultural Crops Research Laboratory, Corvallis, OR
http://www.ars-grin.gov/hcrl/

US Department of Agriculture, Agricultural Research Services, National Clonal Germplasm Repository, Corvallis, OR
http://www.ars-grin.gov/cor/

Wikipedia, the free content encyclopedia
http://en.wikipedia.org/wiki/Main_Page

Other references provided within the chapter

Chapter 3—Wolfberry's Nutrient Profile

References in Chapter 2 are relevant.
Antioxidants Review 2005
http://www.nutraceuticalsworld.com/March05Feature1.htm

Antioxidant Overview, Free Radicals, Oxidative Stress, ORAC Analysis, Brunswick Laboratories Inc.
http://www.brunswicklabs.com/overview_antioxidants.shtml

Assessing berries' health potential, R Wrolstad, Functional Foods and Nutraceuticals, May 2004 issue
http://www.ffnmag.com/NH/ASP/strArticleID/489/strSite/FFNSite/articleDisplay.asp

Blueberries
http://www.whfoods.com/genpage.php?tname=foodspice&dbid=8
http://www.nutritiondata.com/facts-001-02s01ff.html

Center for Food Safety and Applied Nutrition, "CFSAN", US Food and Drug Administration
http://www.cfsan.fda.gov/list.html

Fatty acid composition and antioxidant properties of cold-pressed marionberry, boysenberry, red raspberry and blueberry seed oils. J Parry et al., J. Agric. Food Chem. 2005 Feb 9;53(3):566-73.

Flax seeds
http://www.askdrsears.com/html/4/T041700.asp
http://216.239.63.104/search?q=cache:hggXBmbMHR4J:www.flaxcouncil.ca/FlaxPrimer_Chptr12.pdf+flax+nutrients&hl=en
http://www.ecochem.com/flax_facts.html
http://www.nutritiondata.com/facts-001-02s02fv.html

Functional Foods, G Mazza (Editor), 1998, CRC Press, ISBN 1566764874

HealthCastle Nutrition Information
http://www.healthcastle.com/food_supplements.shtml

Just Say NO (nitric oxide), LJ Ignarro
http://www.research.ucla.edu/chal/25.htm

The role of leucine in weight loss diets and glucose homeostasis. DK Layman, J Nutr. 2003; 133:261S-267S

Linus Pauling Institute, Micronutrient Information Center, Oregon State University, Corvallis
http://lpi.oregonstate.edu/infocenter/index.html
Natural Food Hub
http://www.naturalhub.com/natural_food_guide_fruit_common.htm

Ningxia Wolfberry Collection, Bai Shouning (Editor), Ningxia Peoples Publisher, 1998, ISBN 722702030

NO More Heart Disease, LJ Ignarro, St Martin's Press, 2005, ISBN 0312335814

NutritionData
http://www.nutritiondata.com/index.html

Nutrition Fact Sheets, Feinberg School of Medicine, Northwestern University, 2005 http://www.feinberg.northwestern.edu/nutrition/fact-sheets.html

Omega-3 Fatty Acids and Health. JA Nettleton, Chapman and Hall, 1995, ISBN 0412988615

Papaya: The Healthy Fruit (Natural Health Guide), H Tietze, Alive Books, 2002, ISBN 1553120051

Papaya
http://www.whfoods.com/genpage.php?tname=foodspice&dbid=47
http://www.bawarchi.com/health/papaya.html#pap-nutri
http://www.nutritiondata.com/facts-001-02s01j5.html

Phytochemical composition and pigment stability of acai (Euterpe oleracea Mart.). D Del Pozo-Insfran, CH Brenes, ST Talcott, J Agric Food Chem 2004, 52:1539-1545

Polyphenols, R Sahelian
http://www.raysahelian.com/polyphenols.html

Reactive oxygen species, aging, and antioxidant nutraceuticals, J Lee, N Koo, DB Min, Comprehen Rev Food Sci Food Safety 2004, 3:21-33

Rich Nature Nutraceutical Labs
http://www.richnature.com

Role of the arginine-nitric oxide pathway in the regulation of vascular smooth muscle cell proliferation. LJ Ignarro , GM Buga, LW Wei, PM Bauer, G Wu, P del Soldato, Proc Natl Acad Sci 2001, 98:4202-4208

Separation procedures for naturally occurring antioxidant phytochemicals, R Tsao, Z Deng, J Chromatog B 2004, 812:85-99

Spinach and Beyond: Loving Life and Dark Green Leafy Vegetables, LD Feldt, Moon Field, 2003, ISBN 0965213218

Spinach
http://www.whfoods.com/genpage.php?tname=foodspice&dbid=43
http://www.wholehealthmd.com/refshelf/foods_view/1,1523,35,00.html#Nutrition_Chart

The Flax Cookbook: Recipes and Strategies for Getting the Most from the Most Powerful Plant on the Planet, E Magee, Marlowe Publishers, 2003, ISBN 156924507X

USDA Database for the Flavonoid Content of Selected Foods, 2003 http://www.nal.usda.gov/fnic/foodcomp/Data/Flav/flav.pdf

World's Healthiest Foods
http://www.whfoods.com/

Young Living Essential Oils, Berry Young Juice, Wolfberries, Science, http://berryyoungjuice.com/wolfberries.jsp
http://berryyoungjuice.com/science.jsp

Chapter 4—Wolfberry Signature Nutrient: Polysaccharides

Cellular and physiological effects of Ganoderma lucidum (Reishi). D Sliva, Mini-Rev Med Chem 2004, 4:873-879

Immune receptors for polysaccharides from Ganoderma lucidum. BM Shao, H Dai, W Xu, ZB Lin, XM Gao, Biochem Biophys Res Comm 2004, 323:133-141

Nondigestible oligo—and polysaccharides (dietary fiber): their physiology and role in human health and food. BC Tungland, D Meyer, Comprehen Rev Food Sci Food Safety 2002, 1:73-92

Resistant starches and health. CW Kendall, A Emam, LS Augustin, DJ Jenkins, J AOAC Int 2004, 87:769-774

Whole grains and human health, J Slavin, Nutr Res Rev 2004, 17:99-110

Why whole grains are protective: biological mechanisms. J Slavin. Proc Nutr Soc 2003, 62:129-134

Chapter 5—Wolfberry Signature Nutrient: Carotenoids

Carotenoids and flavonoids in organically grown spinach (Spinacia oleracea L) genotypes after deep frozen storage. U Kidmose, P Knuthsen, M Edelenbos, U Justesen, E Hegelund, J Sci Food Agric, 2001, 81:918-923

Carotenoids In Health And Disease (Oxidative Stress and Disease), NJ Krinsky et al. (Editors), 2004, Marcel Dekker Publishers, ISBN 0824754166

Eye Health Update, Y Naguib, Nutraceuticals World, May 2005, 46-55

Lipophilic and hydrophilic antioxidant capacities of common foods in the United States. X Wu, GR Beecher, JM Holden, DB Haytowitz, SE Gebhardt, RL Prior, J Agric Food Chem 2004 Jun 16;52(12):4026-37

Macular Degeneration: The Complete Guide to Saving and Maximizing Your Sight, Mogk LG, Mogk M, revised edition, NY: Ballantine Books, 2003, ISBN 0345457110

Reactive oxygen species, aging and antioxidative nutraceuticals, J Lee, N Koo, DB Min, Comprehen Rev Food Sci Food Safety 2003, 3:21-33

Other references provided within the chapter

Chapter 6—Wolfberry Nutrient and Disease Research: Implied Benefits

References in Chapters 2 and 3 are relevant

Other references provided within the chapter

Chapter 7—Wolfberries and Traditional Chinese Medicine (TCM)

Classics of Traditional Chinese Medicine from the US National Library of Medicine, History of Medicine Division, National Institutes of Health, Bethesda http://www.nlm.nih.gov/hmd/chinese/chinesehome.html

Hanlin Academy, TCM and Wolfberries
http://www.hanlin.hit.bg/wolfberry.htm

History of Traditional Chinese Medicine, Karolinska Institute Library, Stockholm,
http://www.mic.ki.se/China.html

Practical Therapeutics of Traditional Chinese Medicine, Y Wu, W Fischer, J Fratkin (Editors) 1997, Paradigm, ISBN 0912111399

The Shambhala Guide to Traditional Chinese Medicine, D Reid, Shambhala, 1996, ISBN 1570621411

The Essential Book of Traditional Chinese Medicine, L Yanchi et al.,1988, Columbia Univ. Press, ISBN 0231103573

When east meets west: the relationship between yin-yang and antioxidation-oxidation. B Ou, D Huang, M Hampsch-Woodill, JA Flanagan, FASEB J 2003, 17:127-9

Chapter 8—Botanical Taxonomy for Wolfberry

Highbush Blueberry Fact Sheet, Oregon State University, Corvallis
http://berrygrape.oregonstate.edu/fruitgrowing/berrycrops/blueberry/blueplnt.htm

International Code of Botanical Nomenclature
http://www.bgbm.fu-berlin.de/iapt/nomenclature/code/SaintLouis/0027Ch3Sec4a023.htm

Oregon's Raspberries and Blackberries
http://www.oregon-berries.com/cx1/cx1.htm

Plants for a Future, Lycium barbarum
http://www.ibiblio.org/pfaf/cgi-bin/arr_html?Lycium+barbarum&CAN=COMIND

Studies on Lycium barbarum [in Chinese], B Shouning, 1999, China Scientific Book Services
http://www.hceis.com/book.asp?id=1346

US Highbush Blueberry Council
http://www.ushbc.org/

Wild Blueberry Association of North America, WBANA
http://www.wbana.org/

Chapter 9—Wolfberry Cultivation, Harvesting and Geography

China Geography
http://worldfacts.us/China-geography.htm
China Map
http://worldfacts.us/China-map.htm

Maps and Geographical Features of Chinese Provinces and Autonomous Regions http://www.paulnoll.com/China/Provinces/

Ningxia on Encyclopedia.com
http://www.encyclopedia.com/html/N/NingxiaH1.asp

Ningxia
http://sacu.org/ningxia.html
http://www.suite101.com/article.cfm/east_asian_history/112677
http://www.cpirc.org.cn/en/30Province1999-ningxia.htm
http://www.china.org.cn/e-xibu/2JI/3JI/ningxia/ningxia-ban.htm
http://www.unescap.org/esid/psis/population/database/chinadata/ningxia.htm

Xinjiang
http://www.encyclopedia.com/html/x/xinjiang.asp

Yellow River, geography and history, University of Massachusetts, Dartmouth, http://www.cis.umassd.edu/~gleung/geofo/geogren.html

Yellow River Conservancy Commission
http://www.yellowriver.gov.cn/eng/

Chapter 10—Processing Effects on Wolfberry Nutrients

Effects of cooking, processing, storage, http://www.whfoods.com/genpage.php?tname=nutrient&dbid=116

Antioxidants in raspberry: on-line analysis links antioxidant activity to a diversity of individual metabolites. J Beekwilder, H Jonker, P Meesters, RD Hal, IM van der Meer, CH Ric de Vos. J Agric Food Chem 2005 May 4;53(9):3313-20.

Effect of ascorbic acid and dehydration on concentrations of total phenolics, antioxidant capacity, anthocyanins, and color in fruits. TM Rababah, KI Ereifej, L Howard, J Agric Food Chem 2005 Jun 1;53(11):4444-7

Other references provided within the chapter

BACK COVER

"Flowering in Warm Spring", 1997, ink on xuan paper by Ms. Xu Shulin, wife of Dr. Cui Yueli (see Dedication), mother of Dr. Xiaoping Zhang (book co-author), former Director of the Beijing Opera, now living in Beijing.

Bottom left, wolfberries being picked on Rich Nature's farm in Zhongning County, Ningxia, China; center, bagged wolfberry harvest before screening and grading of fruit; right, dried wolfberries.

Made in the USA